Clinical Essays in
Obstetrics and Gynaecology
for
MRCOG Part II
(And Other Postgraduate Exams)

Clinical Essays in Obstetrics and Gynaecology for MRCOG Part II
(And Other Postgraduate Exams)

Second Edition

Seema Sharma
MRCOG MD DGO
Consultant Obstetrician and Gynaecologist
New Delhi, India
drseemagyn@hotmail.com

Mala Arora
FRCOG (UK) FICOG FICMCH DA (UK)
Chairperson FOGSI Quiz Committee
Faridabad, Haryana, India
malanarinder@gmail.com

Foreword
Anthony Hollingworth

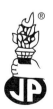

JAYPEE BROTHERS MEDICAL PUBLISHERS (P) LTD
New Delhi • Panama City • London

Published by
Jaypee Brothers Medical Publishers (P) Ltd

Corporate Office
4838/24 Ansari Road, Daryaganj, **New Delhi** 110002, India
Phone: +91-11-43574357, Fax: +91-11-43574314
Website: www.jaypeebrothers.com

Offices in India
- **Ahmedabad**, e-mail: ahmedabad@jaypeebrothers.com
- **Bengaluru**, e-mail: bangalore@jaypeebrothers.com
- **Chennai**, e-mail: chennai@jaypeebrothers.com
- **Delhi**, e-mail: jaypee@jaypeebrothers.com
- **Hyderabad**, e-mail: hyderabad@jaypeebrothers.com
- **Kochi**, e-mail: kochi@jaypeebrothers.com
- **Kolkata**, e-mail: kolkata@jaypeebrothers.com
- **Lucknow**, e-mail: lucknow@jaypeebrothers.com
- **Mumbai**, e-mail: mumbai@jaypeebrothers.com
- **Nagpur**, e-mail: nagpur@jaypeebrothers.com

Overseas Offices
- **Central America Office, Panama City, Panama,** Ph: 001-507-317-0160,
  e-mail: cservice@jphmedical.com, Website: www.jphmedical.com
- **Europe Office, UK,** Ph: +44 (0) 2031708910, e-mail: info@jpmedpub.com

Clinical Essays in Obstetrics and Gynaecology for MRCOG Part II (And Other Postgraduate Exams)

First Edition: 2007
Second Edition: **2011**
ISBN 978-93-5025-388-5
Typeset at JPBMP typesetting unit
Printed at Rajkamal Electric Press, Plot No. 2, Phase-IV, Kundli, Haryana.

Dedicated to

*Late Prof Ram Avtar Maini and my parents
Amrit and Santosh Maini*

Foreword

I am delighted to be able to write a foreword for the second edition of the book *Clinical Essays in Obstetrics and Gynaecology for MRCOG Part II (And Other Postgraduate Exams)*. My previous foreword is as applicable with this book as it was for the last.

Preparing for any examination can be a daunting task. It is paramount when studying for the MRCOG part II examination, that no area of the curriculum be omitted. The MRCOG examination continues to evolve and the extended matching questions (EMQs) are now becoming an equal part of the exam. However, an essay component is being maintained and this book addresses a wide range of questions which are relevant for the exam. The essay plans are very comprehensive and provide an excellent way of consolidating knowledge about the various topics. It is important to remember that this exam is aimed at someone who is in their third specialist registrar year and so a general rather than a subspecialist knowledge is what is required in order to proceed through this part of the exam to the OSCEs.

Anthony Hollingworth
MB ChB (Manchester) MBA (Keele)
PhD (London) FRCS (Ed) FRCOG
Consultant in Obstetrics and Gynaecology
Whipps Cross University Hospital Trust
London

Preface

It gives us great pleasure and satisfaction to bring out the second edition of this book. Keeping in mind the changed format of the MRCOG examination, we have modified and updated the presentation of essays to make it more reader friendly. Beside MRCOG, postgraduate students appearing for Diploma, National Board and MD Examinations may find it useful.

Important points for the general understanding, MCQs and EMQs have been incorporated at the end of each essay and all possible care has been taken to verify the accuracy of course content. Your suggestions to improve the book in any form are welcome.

Seema Sharma
drseemagyn@hotmail.com
Mala Arora
malanarinder@gmail.com

Acknowledgements

We thank Mr Anthony Hollingworth for supporting us selflessly for this project. He has provided clarity of thought and content all along, despite his extremely hectic schedule.

My children, Hriday and Niyati and my husband Sandeep have all been very understanding and patient with me while I was busy with the book. They have encouraged me and showered me with unconditional love and affection. Thank you for being there for me.

Thank you, Dr Mala for being such a lovely person and for pushing me to do things better. It has been a pleasure to be associated with you for this project.

Contents

TIPS for MRCOG Part II Examination

MRCOG is a UK based exam. You need to read their books and guidelines and answer questions as if you are in a UK hospital. Some situations may be peculiar to that part of the world and one should accept and prepare oneself accordingly.

Enroll in the trainees register and visit the RCOG website frequently. Read all the guidelines and statements issued by the college, including the NICE, FFPRC guidelines and CEMACH reports.

Read as many SAQ books as possible. It is best to attempt at least one question per day in stipulated time, but if that is not possible at least go through the text in your free time. It familiarises the student with the important course content and decreases the possibility of encountering the unknown at the time of final examination.

Make your own list of common percentages from the guidelines and other text on the RCOG website. List of autosomal dominant and recessive conditions, survival at key gestational ages, and at various stages of malignancies can be prepared. Keep this list handy and refer to it frequently so that it can be used in essay questions to support your arguments and in multiple choice questions.

It helps to stay calm. Practice some kind of meditation, deep breathing or exercise regimen.

At least two weeks prior to the examination date, set your body rhythm according to the examination timetable in your country. In India the exam usually starts at noon and goes on till late evening. Practice the essays, MCQs and EMQs as if in actual exam situation.

Learn to incorporate certain terms in your essays, the politically correct words as they say;
- Multidisciplinary treatment
- Information leaflets/ written information to the woman
- Additional counselling whenever the couple requires
- Informed decision by the woman, sympathetic and non-judgmental attitude
- Anti-D whenever applicable in a nonsensitised rhesus negative woman
- Treatment according to hospital protocols
- Refer to specialist care or tertiary set up, involve support groups

- Some women may be normal with a given condition and may require only reassurance.
- Clear documentation of the counselling session/procedure/woman's wishes in the case notes whenever the question demands.
- Folic acid to be started.
- Breastfeeding is not contraindicated (except HIV, phenylketonuria, lactose intolerance in baby)
- Skills and drills in all obstetric emergencies with continued professional development.
- Pregnancy test wherever relevant.
- Always try and add the 3 C.... *Chlamydia* screening, cervical smear, contraception advice.

I would like to recommend that the student just scribbles these phrases onto the rough sheet and add whatever is required in each question according to the situation. This may add a few extra marks and thus prove invaluable to the borderline candidates.

Additional tips for formulating the short essays...

Read the question 2-3 times and establish what is being asked. Do not be in a hurry to show your expertise on the topic. Underline the key words if you like. Remember that these details especially the ones about age, parity and life-style are there for a reason and plan your answers accordingly. Pain abdomen in the early first trimester, i.e. 6 to 8 weeks is more likely to be ectopic, 24 weeks is the legal age of viability in UK, 25 years is the start of cervical screening programme in UK,34 weeks after which antenatal steroids are no longer recommended, 38 weeks is fetal maturity, 41 weeks at which induction of labour is beneficial. Ask yourself why this information is there and what is more likely to happen at this time or to a woman of this parity.

Think straight. They are asking you about everyday things that you have done and experienced before. Think of all possible angles—related to the patient, her relatives, and medical personnel in that particular situation.

Start with simple straight forward physiological things first. Do not doubt the intentions of the examiner. Usually there are no hidden complexities in a question. If the question asks about the management of premature rupture of membranes, do not waste space by trying to establish whether leaking is actually present or not. Assume it is the correct diagnosis. If you feel very strongly about first establishing the correct diagnosis, you may mention in a line that you would like to reconfirm the diagnosis and then start the answer.

Plan your answer and jot down important points that you will incorporate in a rough sheet. Jot down whatever comes to your mind regarding that scenario and then finally select while writing the final answer. Sometimes even fleeting thoughts are important and if we do not put it in a rough sheet we forget it later because of the exam stress.

Never leave a question unanswered. One short answer question is likely to be out of the blue but remember it is difficult for everyone. Do not panic and think how you can maximize your scores. Even if you mention a few important points, you may score a few marks which can make a difference for the borderline candidates.

One can ask for extra rough sheets during the exam but not the actual answer sheets. So use the space judiciously. People with big print handwriting may have a disadvantage.

Write in short, simple sentences with legible handwriting. You will not get marked, if the examiner cannot read what you have written. Usually there is no need for underlining. Avoid repetitions in various forms. Do not get sidetracked while writing and start adding subheadings to the highlighted point. It is important to give the global picture and incorporate all the important points before one runs out of space.

The space provided for the answers is limited, so memorize some space savers like;
• Medical optimization prior to surgery
• A risk and need assessment at booking with individualized flexible care plan
• Woman's wishes and her viewpoints should be considered, etc.

When there is a question about counselling, describe the risks and benefits of your options. Informed consent from the patient is essential.

Diagnosis usually involves history, examination and appropriate investigations. Management involves diagnosis, medical, surgical and supportive treatment.

Plan of care for a pregnant woman starts with antenatal assessment (including foetal and maternal monitoring), and includes intrapartum management (including mode of delivery); postpartum care (including advice on breastfeeding- if relevant), contraception and preconception counselling for the next pregnancy. Start from head to toe and from start to finish for a procedure.

Revise your answers towards the end when you are in a more balanced state of mind.

Time table for the MRCOG Part II exam

Short Answer Question (SAQ)	4	30% of total marks
Multiple Choice Question (MCQ)	240	30% of total marks
Extended Matching Question (EMQ)	90	40% of total marks

The revised format will entail candidates sitting three papers on the day of the Part II written examination:

Paper 1 (4 SAQs) – 105 minutes
Paper 2 (120 MCQs, 45 EMQs) – 135 minutes
Paper 3 (120 MCQs, 45 EMQs) – 135 minutes

Time allowed: 1.45 hours   *MM 80*

1. A 23-year-old primigravida presents at 16 weeks for her booking visit. She has a body weight of 140 kg and a body mass index of 40. She has no other apparent risk factor.   (14, 6 marks)
   a. What specific problems would you anticipate during the course of this pregnancy?
   b. What advice would you give her regarding her weight and associated management during pregnancy?

2. Mrs. Quincy is unable to pass urine even 8 hours after her vaginal delivery. She has had an uneventful outlet forceps for assistance.   (8, 6, 6 marks)
   a. Enumerate the principles of her management.
   b. One liter of urine was drained on catheterisation. Outline her subsequent management.
   c. What steps should be taken in her next pregnancy to prevent recurrence?

3. You are the SpR on emergency duty and you have just been informed that the SHO on duty has created a uterine perforation while performing a Medical Termination of Pregnancy.   (6, 9, 5 marks)
   a. What is your initial assessment of the case on reaching the operation theatre?
   b. How will you manage the case in theatre?
   c. Outline your post- operative management of the case.

4. An 18-year-old woman presents at A and E. She is terrified and anxious and reveals that she has been sexually assaulted by her boyfriend. She does not wish to inform the police as yet. You are the OB/GYN registrar on emergency duty.   (6, 6, 8 marks)
   a. What relevant facts should be kept in mind before you examine her?
   b. How will you examine and investigate her?
   c. How will you manage her condition?

1. **A 23-year-old primigravida presents at 16 weeks for her booking visit. She has a body weight of 140 kg and a body mass index of 40. She has no other apparent risk factor.**

a. **What specific problems would you anticipate during the course of this pregnancy?** **(14 marks)**

Antepartum: Hypertensive disorders, gestational diabetes, thromboembolism and urinary tract infection are common in obese women. 2 marks

Maternal blood pressure is difficult to determine when the upper arm is fat. Large and appropriate sized cuffs should be used to prevent falsely high reading. 1 mark

As the pregnancy proceeds it may be difficult to evaluate the size of foetus, presenting part, liquor estimation and foetal heart sounds by conventional means. Serial ultrasound scans may be required to evaluate foetal growth. Ultrasonic foetal weight assessments may be unreliable if too much adipose tissue in abdominal wall hampers visualisation. 2 marks

Intrapartum: During labour it may be mechanically difficult to site an intravenous cannula or an epidural catheter. Involvement of a senior obstetrician and anaesthetist is desirable for delivery, airway management, and analgesia. Vigilance for thrombophlebitis should be maintained. 2 marks

Intrapartum monitoring may be difficult. Internal monitoring with foetal scalp electrodes is more appropriate. 1 mark

There may be poor progress of labour because of persistently high head and occipito-posterior position due to excessive fat in ischiorectal fossa. 1 mark

Postpartum haemorrhage, low apgar scores, foetal macrosomia and shoulder dystocia are commonly associated. 1 mark

If caesarean section is required, both surgery and anaesthesia is more hazardous. Regional analgesia should be preferred over general anaesthesia. 1 mark

Delayed wound healing due to sweating, haematoma formation and diabetes is common. Single layer wound closure with nonabsorbable sutures is preferable. Placement of prophylactic surgical drains at wound site is debatable. 1 mark

Deep vein thrombosis is more common in obese women. 1 mark

Neonate should be monitored for signs of hypoglycaemia. 1 mark

b. **What advice would you give her regarding her weight and associated management during pregnancy?** **(6 marks)**

Pregnancy is not the time for weight loss or extensive dietary restrictions. There is no role of bariatric surgeries during pregnancy. 1 mark

She should take up an appointment with the dietician and be on a weight maintenance regimen. The ideal weight gain for her during pregnancy should be 8 to 9 kg. 1 mark

After delivery early ambulation, TED stockings, and prophylactic heparin should be considered. 1 mark

Encourage early breastfeeding as the foetus may be more prone to hypoglycaemia. 1 mark

Adequate contraception before next pregnancy in the form of barriers, or intrauterine devices should be prescribed. Combined oral pills are a relative contraindication. 1 mark

She should be encouraged to lose weight before next pregnancy. 1 mark

IMPORTANT INFORMATION

Obesity is showing a globally increasing trend. Twenty percent women were found to be obese according to 2003 to 2005 CEMACH studies in UK.

Divide the problems into ante-partum, intra-partum and post-partum period. BMI values (weight in kg/height in m^2) are interpreted as follows:

BMI	Interpretation	Recommended weight gain in pregnancy
< 15	Emaciation	
15–20	Underweight	12.5–18 kg
20–25	Desirable weight	11.5–16 kg
25–30	Overweight	7–11.5 kg
30 and above	Serious obesity	5–9 kg

Women with BMI between 30 to 35 are moderately obese while those with BMI more than 35 are morbidly obese.

During preconception counselling advise a woman regarding:

1. Risk of falling pregnant with their current weight.

2. Possible lifestyle measures to ensure sustained weight loss and improve fertility.

3. *Identify potential complications due to obesity which may compromise maternal and foetal outcome.*

4. *Advice commencement of folic acid 5 mg/day.*

5. *Advice commencement of 10 μg of vitamin D/day.*

Obesity increases the risk of congenital malformations and increases both long-term and short-term perinatal mortality as an independent risk factor. There is said to be a 30 percent increase in overall adult mortality with every 5 kg/m^2 increase in BMI.

Obesity increases the risk of maternal death approximately 4 times. There is a 2-fold increase in neural tube defects esp. spina bifida and still births. There is 1.5 times increase in incidence of cleft palate and lip, cardiovascular and septal defects.

Good asepsis, prophylactic antibiotics and haemostasis should be maintained during delivery.

2. **Mrs Quincy is unable to pass urine even 8 hours after her vaginal delivery. She has had an uneventful outlet forceps for assistance.**

a. **Enumerate the principles of her management.** (8 marks)

Look for risk factors: Ask for history of epidural analgesia, prolonged first and second stage of labour. Primiparity and instrumental delivery are risk factors for voiding dysfunction. 2 marks

Examine the perineum under good light for any possible trauma, lacerations or haematoma. These should be repaired. 2 marks

Provide good analgesia. 1 mark

Catheterise with all aseptic precautions and measure residual urinary volume. Send the mid stream urine sample for analysis and culture. Commence antibiotics if required. 2 marks

Talk to her about the likely cause of urinary retention. Epidural analgesia may blunt the bladder sensation for a variable period. 1 mark

b. **One liter of urine was drained on catheterisation. Outline her subsequent management.** (6 marks)

Insert indwelling urinary catheter for 24 hours. If on removal she is unable to void within 6 hours, measure urinary volume by bladder ultrasound. If urine volume is more than 500 ml, keep the catheter for one week. 2 marks

Commence antibiotics, if not done before. 1 mark

Multidisciplinary input may be required by an anaesthetist and urologist. 1 mark

Persistent voiding dysfunction beyond two weeks requires neurological assessment and intermittent self-catheterisation. 2 marks

c. **What steps should be taken in her next pregnancy to prevent recurrence?** (6 marks)

Measure voiding volume and residual urine by ultrasound once during her antenatal period. If residual urine is $\geq$ 150 ml, refer her to an urogynaecologist. 1 mark

Encourage adequate fluid intake and regular voiding once in 4 to 6 hours during labour. Avoid constipation during late pregnancy and labour. 2 marks

Document all voiding events during labour and keep output record.   1 mark

Prompt catheterisation and early recognition of dysfunction is important. If already catheterised, the bulb should be deflated during the second stage to avoid possible damage.   2 marks

3. **You are the SpR on emergency duty and you have just been informed that the SHO on duty has created a uterine perforation while performing a Medical Termination of Pregnancy.**

   a. **What is your initial assessment of the case on reaching the operation theatre?** **(6 marks)**

Scrub and join the team. Elicit a short history from the SHO—gestational age/ uterine size/likely instrument of perforation/approximate blood loss.   1 mark

Inform the anaesthetist for intubation/theatre nurse to prepare for a laparoscopy and possible laparotomy.   1 mark

Enquire about vital parameters to assess the blood loss. Send blood for cross match and clotting studies.   1 mark

Replace blood and fluids appropriately.   1 mark

Foley's to be inserted to empty the bladder and measure urinary output.   1 mark

Perform a speculum and vaginal examination to ascertain active blood loss and uterine size.   1 mark

   b. **How will you manage the case in theatre?** **(9 marks)**

Inform Obstetrics/Gynaecology consultant on call.   1 mark

Proceed with laparoscopic examination—assess damage to uterus/bowel/bladder.   2 marks

Complete MTP under laparoscopic vision.   1 mark

Small perforation and no injury to neighbouring organs—manage expectantly; add antibiotics and oxytocics.   2 marks

If active bleeding/big perforation/injury elsewhere are seen, proceed to laparotomy to repair damage. Check haemostasis before closure. Call surgeon if required.   2 marks

In a profusely bleeding perforation, hysterectomy may be required. Add thromboprophylaxis.   1 mark

   c. **Outline your post-operative management of the case.** **(5 marks)**

Complete theatre notes meticulously.   1 mark

Clinical Risk Management (CRM) forms to be filled.   1 mark

Debrief the patient when she is comfortable and answer all her queries honestly.

1 mark

Reassess her need for thromboprophylaxis.

1 mark

Inform her consultant and GP about the incident and arrange follow-up visits to discuss contraception before discharge.

1 mark

4. **An 18-year-old presents at A and E. She is terrified and anxious and reveals that she has been sexually assaulted by her boyfriend. She does not wish to inform the police as yet. You are the OB/GYN registrar on emergency duty.**

a. **What relevant facts should be kept in mind before you examine her?**
(6 marks)

As a competent adult she has a choice whether to involve the police or not.
2 marks

Put her at ease and maintain her dignity at all times. Inform her that she has a right to refuse any part of examination.
1 mark

Record all information about the assault and keep separate from clinical notes. Show her these notes which can be utilised should she change her mind later on.
1 mark

All relevant samples should be collected and preserved according to the hospital policy. She should be informed that if she chooses not to involve the police within a stipulated time, these samples would be destroyed and written consent taken for the same.
2 marks

b. **How will you examine and investigate her?**
(6 marks)

Offer a general physical examination and provide first-aid for minor injuries.
1 mark

Document all injuries/marks/stains.
1 mark

Keep vulval hair and nail clippings/vaginal, oral, and anal swabs according to local hospital protocols. Send endocervical swabs for investigation of Sexually Transmitted Infections (STI). Label and store these in appropriate medium for possible later use.
3 marks

Bag her underclothing after arranging for replacement clothing. Investigate and treat more serious injuries promptly.
1 mark

c. **How will you manage her condition?**
(8 marks)

Encourage her to talk to a supportive friend/ family member.
1 mark

Discuss emergency contraception and offer appropriate choices with 1.5 mg levonorgestrel within 72 hours or copper intrauterine device within 5 days.
2 marks

STI testing should commence as soon as possible and follow-up offered to her. Hepatitis B prophylaxis should be given preferably within 72 hours. 2 marks

Discuss safe accommodation on discharge. Appraise her GP for follow-up and counselling if she consents. 1 mark

Involve a Genitourinary physician if assailant has obvious risk factors for HBV/HIV. Give post-exposure prophylaxis or refer to Genitourinary Medicine (GUM) clinics after 2 weeks. 1 mark

If she refuses to give written consent for police involvement, samples must be destroyed according to hospital policy. 1 mark

Time allowed: 1.45 hours   *MM 80*

1. A 33-years-old woman comes to you for advice as she has noticed a small breast lump on her left breast last week. She is 16 weeks pregnant at present and is very worried as her maternal aunt has recently died of Breast cancer. **(10, 10 marks)**
   a. What is your initial management?
   b. Histology confirms an intraductal carcinoma. She is 20/40 weeks pregnant by now. What is your plan of care for her?

2. A pregnant woman has been referred to you by her GP. She is 11 weeks pregnant and has 2 children, 6 months and 5 years; at home. She is still breastfeeding her younger child and her elder one has just been diagnosed with swine flu. **(6, 4, 4, 2, 4 marks)**
   a. She wishes to know more about the disease. What information will you give her?
   b. How will you counsel her about the flu vaccination?
   c. What precautions should she take to protect herself and her younger one from flu?
   d. She wishes to know whether she can continue breastfeeding. What advise will you give her?
   e. She reports to A and E two days later complaining of flu like symptoms. What would be your management?

3. An 8-years-old girl has been referred to the gynAecology OPD with a history of itching in her perineal area. Recently her panties are also getting very dirty by the end of the day. **(8, 12 marks)**
   a. The mother wants to know why this is happening as her daughter has not even started to menstruate.
   b. How will you manage this case?

4. A 28-years-old woman presents at A and E with severe pain in her right breast and malaise. She delivered a healthy baby boy normally 5 days previously. **(7, 7, 6 marks)**
   a. On examination her right breast is tender with prominent veins and her body temperature is 38°C. What is your diagnosis and enumerate the factors responsible for causing it?
   b. How will you treat her?
   c. Two days later she comes back with high-grade fever with chills and unbearable pain in her right breast. She admits that due to the pain she was unable to express milk from her breast. How will you manage her now?

1. **A 33-years-old woman comes to you for advice as she has noticed a small breast lump on her left breast last week. She is 16 weeks pregnant at present and is very worried as her maternal aunt has recently died of breast cancer.**

a. **What is your initial management?** **(10 marks)**

Inform her that 90 per cent of breast lumps are benign. Triple assessment by clinical examination, imaging and cytology is the key to diagnosis.   1 mark

History of associated features like pain, nipple discharge, any previous breast disease, use of combined pills and family history should be asked in detail. (For a familial cancer at least two-first degree relatives should be suffering from it).
                                                                                 2 marks

Examine both the breasts and estimate the size, position, consistency and fixity of lump. Palpate for enlarged axillary and supraclavicular lymph nodes. Physiological changes in breast during pregnancy make clinical examination more difficult and inaccurate.   2 marks

Ultrasound breast will differentiate between solid and cystic lumps.   1 mark

Mammography is safe in pregnancy but contrast enhanced MRI is a better option in dense breasts.   1 mark

Fine needle aspiration cytology or open biopsy may be required for accurate tissue diagnosis. In pregnancy, risk of bleeding, infection or rarely milk fistulas is increased.   1 mark

If the lump is benign it should be left as such and followed after delivery.
                                                                         1 mark

If the lump turns out to be malignant, she should be referred to a specialized oncology set-up.   1 mark

b. **Histology confirms an intraductal carcinoma. She is 20/40 weeks pregnant by now. What is your plan of care for her?** **(10 marks)**

Complete physical examination, haematological investigations and CT chest should be performed. IDC frequently metastasizes to bone, lung, liver or brain. 1 mark

Multidisciplinary treatment with obstetricians, breast surgeons and clinical oncologists is preferred.   1 mark

Have clear discussions with the woman about her treatment. Five year survival in a node negative woman is close to 90 per cent but two-thirds of women have advanced disease at the time of detection.   1 mark

Pregnancy may be continued, as studies have not indicated any long-term survival difference.   1 mark

If she continues with the pregnancy, surgery in the form of lumpectomy/mastectomy with axillary clearance remains the first treatment option, and can be safely performed in the second trimester. Reconstruction can be deferred.

2 marks

Combination chemotherapy with 5FU, Doxorubicin, and cyclophosphamide for 4 to 6 cycles is safe during pregnancy.   1 mark

Avoid radiation but if absolutely essential, use lead shield to decrease the dose received by the fetus.   1 mark

Deliver her at 34 weeks with a caesarean section, after a dose of antenatal steroids.

1 mark

She may safely breastfeed from the unaffected breast if not on any toxic drugs.

1 mark

2. **A pregnant woman has been referred to you by her GP. She is 11 weeks pregnant and has 2 children, 6 months and 5 years; at home. She is still feeding her younger child and her elder one has just been diagnosed with swine flu.**

a. **She wishes to know more about the disease. What information will you give her?** **(6 marks)**

Swine flu is a respiratory disease caused by a new strain of flu virus. (H1N1 type A influenza virus). This strain was earlier known to infect pigs (swine family). Since it is a new strain of virus, previously unknown in humans, hence there is no natural immunity as yet. 1 mark

Symptoms are: Fever, cough, shortness of breath and combination of one or many of these: Headache, aching muscles, running nose, sneezing, chills, and tiredness, loss of appetite, vomiting, and diarrhoea. It usually is a mild disease for most people; comes quickly and lasts for one week. 1 mark

In a pregnant woman a swine flu episode may cause miscarriages, preterm delivery and adverse delivery outcomes. Fetal distress and maternal deaths have been reported during labour in complicated cases. Majority of the complications during pregnancy are related to fever which in the first trimester may increase the risk of neural tube and birth defects, and during labour may cause neonatal seizures, encephalopathy, cerebral palsy and fetal death. 2 marks

Certain people like infants, children less than 5 years, pregnant women and immunocompromised individuals; i.e. infected with HIV, any other systemic illness, concurrent respiratory illness are more likely to develop complications. 1 mark

Pregnant women are 6 times more likely to develop serious complications and be hospitalized with swine flu. Teenage mothers and women in their second and third trimesters are at higher-risk. Treatment should be started in all pregnant women suspected to have swine flu without waiting for the lab confirmation. 1 mark

b. **How will you counsel her about the flu vaccination?** **(4 marks)**

Pregnancy is a high-risk condition and NHS offers free preventive swine flu vaccination to all pregnant women. In UK, three different brands of vaccines are available: 1 mark

Pandemrix—Single shot (2 in people less than 10 years), *Celvapan*—at least two shots, 3 weeks apart, and the trivalent Flu shot.

The vaccine is safe in pregnancy, and is well-tolerated. No adverse effects have been noted in women who have conceived immediately after receiving *Pandemrix*. It protects the fetus as well. It may cause mild flu like symptoms up to 48 hr in some people but this is not flu as the vaccine does not have live virus. Some redness, soreness, and swelling at injection site may occur.   1 mark

She needs to vaccinate her children as well, because the usual yearly flu shot given to children or high-risk groups will not protect against swine flu. The vaccine can be combined with other flu vaccines on the same day, but need to be administered in different arms. If a person in high-risk group has had swine flu/taken antivirals before, but has not received vaccine it can still be taken.   1 mark

RCOG recommends Pandemrix in pregnant women because of single dose advantage and higher compliance. The only contraindication to the vaccine is a known allergy to any of the components of the vaccine.   1 mark

c. What precautions should she take to protect herself and her younger one from flu?   4 marks

Swine flu spreads as droplet infection from infected person's oral and nasal secretions. All oronasal secretions should be caught in handkerchiefs/tissues and disposed off properly in bins. Swine flu virus cannot survive outside the human body for long.   1 mark

Keep hard surfaces, infants toys, clean. Household cleansers can reduce the transmission rate.   1 mark

All pregnant women should avoid contact with sick people. If she develops symptoms of flu, she should send a friend (Flu-friend) to collect the medicines from pharmacy.   1 mark

She should be offered chemoprophylaxis with Zanamivir—two inhalations, 5 mg each, once a day for 10 days. In presence of contraindications—Oseltamivir, 75 mg OD for 10 days after the last known exposure. All close contacts of confirmed positive cases should be offered the same.   1 mark

d. She wishes to know whether she can continue breastfeeding. What advice will you give her?   (2 marks)

Viral transmission through breast milk is currently unknown and breastfed infants have a stronger immunity for swine flu. So she should be advised to continue breastfeeding.   1 mark

If she develops active flu, she can express the breast milk in a bottle and a healthy person can feed the baby. Chemoprophylaxis and treatment are not contraindication to breastfeeding.   1 mark

e. She reports to A and E two days later complaining of flu like symptoms. What would be your management? **(4 marks)**

If she already has flu like symptoms she should be offered antiviral treatment as soon as possible to minimise complications. 1 mark

Relenza (Zanamivir) and Tamiflu (oseltamivir) are recommended for pregnant women in an uncomplicated, mild case of swine flu. 1 mark

If the severity of symptoms is more, she should be hospitalised and oseltamivir started. 1 mark

Provide her with National help line no. 08001513100 and information leaflet on "swine flu in pregnancy". 1 mark

IMPORTANT INFORMATION

Acetaminophen is the drug of choice for pyrexia related to H1N1.

Pandemrix is an adjuvanted (ASO₃) vaccine containing Squalene (derived from fish oils), Tocopherol-vit E, Polysorbate 80 and Thiomersal (mercury derivative— but is not harmful in pregnancy). Both vaccines are licensed for use in pregnancy.

Pandemrix is prepared using hen's egg culture. People with a confirmed anaphylaxis/severe reaction to egg products should instead be given celvapan.

For treatment of swine flu Relenza (Zanamivir) is given as inhaler. It is the first choice in pregnancy as systemic absorption and transplacental transfer is minimal. It is given as two inhalations; 5 mg each, twice a day. Both the medications are neuraminidase inhibitors.

Tamiflu (Oseltamivir) is preferred in patients with COPD, who have difficulty in taking inhalers or severely sick people. If a pregnant lady requires hospitalisation, start on oseltamivir. It is given orally, 75 mg BD for 5 days.

RCOG Recommendations

- *All obstetricians, midwives and neonatologists should be encouraged to take the vaccine to protect themselves, their families and their pregnant patients*
- *All pregnant women should be offered the vaccine. This will decrease their chances of contracting the disease and also protect their newborn from swine flu in the neonatal period*
- *Use of face masks will not prevent swine flu. Focus instead on hygiene and clean surroundings*
- *It is safe to consume well cooked pork and pork products*
- *It has issued a travel advirsory to pregnant women against traveling to affected areas.*

3. **An 8-years-old girl has been referred to the gynecology OPD with a history of itching in her perineal area. Recently her panties are also getting very dirty by the end of the day.**

a. **The mother wants to know why this is happening as her daughter has not even started to menstruate.** **(8 marks)**

Seventy-five per cent of vaginal discharge in children is nonspecific.   1 mark

Infection, presence of foreign body, pin worm infection, child abuse and rarely tumours could be the reason.   3 marks

If the discharge is itchy, offensive and is staining her panties to make her uncomfortable, she needs treatment.   1 mark

It should be explained that children are exposed to more bacteria due to their play habits, lack of estrogen and their vagina has a neutral pH which offers poor resistance to bacteria. Vagina of young girls also lack glycogen, lactobacilli (good bacteria) and sufficient antibodies which make it difficult to remove harmful germs in the natural way.   2 marks

Poor perineal hygiene can start a scratch-itch- secondary infection cycle which needs to be broken.   1 mark

b. **How will you manage this case?**   **(12 marks)**

The girl should be made to feel comfortable and asked gently about the nature, and color of discharge along with the course of progression of the problem.
     1 mark

For examination, anaesthesia may be required. Use Huffman vaginoscope or test tube with otoscope, but not otoscope alone. Take special care to avoid injury if nasal speculum is used.   1 mark

If any foreign body is visible, it should be removed by small swab or irrigation. Knee chest position is helpful during the procedure.   1 mark

Maintenance of good perineal hygiene should be stressed.   1 mark

She should avoid bubble baths, soft soap and swimming till she gets well.
     1 mark

If there is evidence of infection, cultures should be obtained from vulva and peri-anal area. Only 25 per cent of cultures will identify the causative organism.
     1 mark

For severe irritation, sitz baths and broad spectrum antibiotics may be required for 10 to 14 days. Treat her for pinworm infection. 2 marks

Child abuse is a possibility and this aspect should be taken up with the girl and her mother. 2 marks

If itching is intense, a combination of antifungal and 0.5 per cent hydrocortisone cream should be given for vulval application. 2 marks

4. A 28-years-old woman presents at A and E with severe pain in her right breast and malaise. She delivered a healthy baby boy normally 5 days previously.

a. On examination her right breast is tender with prominent veins and her body temperature is 38°C. What is your diagnosis and enumerate the factors responsible for causing it?   (7 marks)

Puerperal mastitis is the likely diagnosis.   1 mark

It is most commonly seen in early puerperium due to failure to empty the breast adequately.   1 mark

Fissuring of nipples and bacterial inoculation from infant's mouth and mother's skin and lowered maternal immune defenses play a role.   2 marks

Poor nipple and skin care allows it to crack easily.   1 mark

Incorrect position of the infant for nursing causes nipple cracking and bleeding.
                    2 marks

b. How will you treat her?   (7 marks)

She should continue nursing as the infection is extraductal. If unable to do so, breast milk must be emptied with the help of breast pump.   1 mark

Explain to her the right position for baby's latching.   2 marks

Mother should maintain adequate hydration and apply moist heat on the breast (warm towels) to help good milk expulsion.   2 marks

NSAIDs to be started for pain relief.   1 mark

Start empirical antibiotics—Dicloxacillin/ampicillin/erythromycin/cephalexin.
                    1 mark

d. Two days later she comes back with high-grade fever with chills and unbearable pain in her right breast. She admits that due to the pain she was unable to express milk from her breast. How will you manage her now?   (6 marks)

Persistent infection along with inadequate emptying has led to breast abscess.
                    1 mark

Cease nursing on the affected side. Send milk cultures after discarding the first 3 cc.   2 marks

Commence intravenous antibiotics—ampicillin 1 g IV, 6 h with clindamycin 900 mg IV 8 hours or metronidazole 500 mg IV 6 hours.   1 mark

Absence of favourable response within 48 to 72 hours requires surgical I and D.
                                                                        2 marks

Time allowed: 1.45 hours   *MM 80*

1. a. Enumerate the etiology and consequences of vaginal childbirth on pelvic floor.   (12, 8 marks)
   b. What preventive strategies should be adopted to contain the damage?

2. An anxious 14 weeks pregnant school teacher calls up the hospital to seek advice. One child in her class has been diagnosed to be suffering from varicella.   (7, 6, 7 marks)
   a. Discuss the advice you will give her on telephone.
   b. Three days later you get the information that her VZ IgG is negative and she has started developing the rash. She is worried about the baby and wishes to know the implications.
   c. Discuss the maternal risks and immediate further treatment.

3. A 30-years-old woman has been referred by her GP with a history of previous three consecutive first trimester miscarriages.   (15, 5 marks)
   a. Enumerate and justify your investigations.
   b. Describe the pros and cons of lymphocyte immune therapy.

4. A 15-years-old girl admits to being sexually active. She wishes to use the combined oral contraceptive pills as she has heard a lot about them.
                                          (7, 5, 8 marks)
   a. Highlight the relevant information that you will gather at this consultation.
   b. Discuss the important side effects of OCP's that she needs to know?
   c. She decides to use the OCP's. Discuss the advice that you will give her.

1. a. Enumerate the a etiology and consequences of vaginal childbirth on pelvic floor. **(12 marks)**

Vaginal childbirth is a major precursor of urinary bladder dysfunction, anal incontinence and pelvic organ prolapse. Damage to the perineum is the maximum during first delivery. 2 marks

Prolonged labour, forceps delivery and high birth weight increase the risk of urinary incontinence. Caesarean section reduces the risk, but does not eliminate it as pregnancy itself may weaken the pelvic diaphragm. Non-obstetric factors such as age, obesity and family history are independent factors that confer significant risk of pelvic floor dysfunction. 3 marks

Perineal trauma at the time of vaginal delivery can cause increased incidence of dyspareunia, fistulae and perineal pain in the immediate postpartum period. 1 mark

Mechanical disruption of the pelvic floor and pudendal nerve injury may result in urinary or anal incontinence. Women with inherent weakness of collagen within the pelvic floor are at a higher-risk. 1 mark

Perineal lacerations and episiotomy cause direct injury to pelvic floor. Midline episiotomy is associated with higher disruption of anal sphincter. 2 marks

Muscle trauma secondary to maternal expulsive efforts and descent of foetal head causes a short-term decrease in pelvic floor strength. 1 mark

Nerve damage due to compression effects may cause increased pudendal nerve latency and denervation injury to pubococcygeal and external sphincter muscles. 1 mark

A collagen and connective tissue change during pregnancy and repair of pelvic floor injury with weaker collagen decreases the strength of support mechanisms. 1 mark

b. What preventive strategies should be adopted to contain the damage? **(8 marks)**

Identify "at risk women" during antenatal period. These include women who have stress urinary incontinence prior to conception, history of collagen disorders and those that have experienced previous anal disruption. These women may be offered elective C-section. 2 marks

At the time of delivery, preferably use ventouse over forceps as it is less traumatic to perineum. Avoid difficult vaginal births and use elective caesarean section in selected cases. Use of episiotomy with adequate training of doctors and midwives involved in repair of perineal trauma may decrease morbidity. Women with anal sphincter damage should be recognized early and repaired adequately.

1, 1, 1 mark

Women who develop problems during or after delivery should be offered follow-up with a consultant. Documentation should be meticulous. Every hospital should have their protocols and treatment policies for such women.   2 marks

Education regarding reduction of family size, improved maternal nutrition, pelvic floor exercises, and avoidance of excessive weight gain during pregnancy should be spread. The patient should perform Kegel exercises in the postnatal period.

1 mark

2. **An anxious 14 weeks-pregnant-school teacher calls up the hospital to seek advice. One child in her class has been diagnosed to be suffering from varicella.**

a. **Discuss the advice you will give her on telephone.** **(7 marks)**

Ask about the details of contact history with particular reference to the certainty of infection, number of infected contacts and the degree of exposure especially to vesicular fluid. Enquire about her symptoms and presence of rash.   2 marks

Enquire if she remembers getting varicella in the past, which may suggest immunity.   1 mark

If she has no previous history of varicella, advice her to get her blood varicella zoster IgG titres from stored serum at the time of antenatal booking. The results will be ready in 24 to 48 hours.   1 mark

She should avoid coming to the hospital to prevent contact with other pregnant women and immunocompromised population till the result is known. If she develops any rash or fever while waiting for the results, she should immediately let the health worker know.   1 mark

If she is IgG seropositive, she is immune and should be reassured. Ninety percent of the antenatal population in UK is immune to varicella due to childhood exposure.   1 mark

If the patient is not immune, she may have to be referred to the hospital for VZ immunoglobulins.   1 mark

b. **Three days later you get the information that her VZ IgG is negative and she has started developing the rash. She is worried about the baby and wishes to know the implications.** **(6 marks)**

She should be informed that there is up to 2 percent risk of congenital varicella syndrome (FVS) in the foetus. FVS consists of skin scarring, eye defects, limb hypoplasia, and neurological abnormalities. For this reason the neonate would be examined by ophthalmologist after birth.   2 marks

There is no increase in spontaneous miscarriage rate.   1 mark

A detailed ultrasound should be arranged at 18 to 20 weeks (or after 5 weeks of exposure) to detect changes in the foetus.   2 marks

Foetal blood sampling to demonstrate varicella IgM in suspicious foetuses can be offered if parents are very anxious and are willing to accept the risks of cordocentesis and termination.   1 mark

c. Discuss the maternal risks and immediate further treatment. (7 marks)

Varicella in adults is rare but has a higher morbidity.   1 mark

One in ten affected women may develop pneumonia, hepatitis or encephalitis with a severe infection.   1 mark

After the development of rash V-Z immune globulin is of no use.   1 mark

Oral acyclovir should be started as soon as possible after an informed consent at 800 mg five times a day for seven days. This decreases the severity of infection and prevents complications.   2 marks

She should be advised to come immediately to the hospital if she develops breathlessness, headaches, visual problems, abnormal bleeding from anywhere or a dense rash.   2 marks

IMPORTANT NOTE

The incubation period of chicken pox is 14 to 21 days and the period of infectivity is from 48 hours prior to eruption of rash till vesicles crust over in average 6 days.

It is a DNA virus of herpes family and spreads due to droplet infection, fomites, direct contact with vesicular fluid and transplacental transmission.

Eye defects in the foetus can be micropthalmia, chorioretinitis, or cataracts.

Neurological abnormalities can be in the form of microcephaly, cortical atrophy, optic atrophy, bladder and bowel sphincter dysfunction.

3. A 30-year-old woman has been referred by her GP with a history of previous three consecutive first trimester miscarriages.

a. Enumerate and justify your investigations. (15 marks)

A couple with recurrent pregnancy losses may have more than one aetiological factor responsible for the miscarriages. Hence the following investigations need to be carried out in all patients. 1 mark

Genetic Causes 2 marks

Peripheral blood karyotyping for both the partners. Three to five percent of couples may be carriers of balanced translocations in one of the partners.

Perform karyotyping of products of conception in case of any future miscarriage.

Anatomical Causes 2 marks

TVS, preferably 3-D ultrasound will pick up uterine anomalies and cervical incompetence. These anomalies are more likely to cause a mid-trimester loss but these should be corrected before the next conception.

Sonohysterography, or Hysterosalpingography and/or Hysteroscopy should be performed in select cases. Hysteroscopy will also provide the opportunity to correct a septate uterus, remove submucous fibroids and endometrial polyps and divide intrauterine adhesions.

Antiphospholipid Syndrome (APL) 2 marks

The prevalence of these antibodies is 15 percent in patients with recurrent miscarriages as compared to 2 percent in fertile women.

Two positive tests (six weeks apart) for either lupus anticoagulant (by dilute Russell's viper venom time (dRVVT) test) or anticardiolipin (aCL) antibodies of IgG and/or IgM class present in medium or high titer are diagnostic for APL.

Infective Causes 2 marks

Both the partners should be screened for genital tract infections like chlamydia, genital tuberculosis (for Asian immigrants), and bacterial vaginosis.

Testing for TORCH infections is not advised as this group is only implicated in sporadic miscarriages and not for recurrent miscarriages.

Hormonal Causes 4 marks

Polycystic Ovaries are associated with early miscarriages especially if associated with hyperandrogenemia and/or hyperinsulinaemia.

Hyperprolactinemia is primarily related with infertility but may also cause miscarriages due to corpus luteal dysfunction.

Autoimmune thyroiditis is associated with a higher incidence of miscarriages.

Premature ovarian failure with FSH levels more than 20 will result in early miscarriages due to aging oocytes.

Thrombophilias   *2 marks*

Inherited thrombophilias result in a thrombogenic state which results in recurrent miscarriages.

She should be tested for Factor V Leiden mutation, activated Protein C resistance, Protein S deficiency, Antithrombin 3 deficiency, and Methyl tetrahydrofolate Reductase (MTFHR) gene mutation.

b. Describe the pros and cons of lymphocyte immune therapy.   (5 marks)

If all the relevant investigations for RPL are normal, the patient is classified as having unexplained recurrent miscarriages or alloimmune causes.

Leukocyte Immune Therapy (LIT) involves injection of leukocytes from the husband or a third party donor in the mother in order to alleviate the alloimmune causes of recurrent miscarriages.   2 marks

The benefits of LIT are not clearly proven in patients with unexplained recurrent miscarriages. A Cochrane review that reviewed thirteen studies concluded that LIT therapy is no better than placebo in unexplained recurrent miscarriages.
                                                                        1 mark

The procedure carries the risk of transmitting communicable diseases like HIV, Hepatitis that may be in the window period. It may result in graft versus host reaction and Foetal Autoimmune Thrombocytopenia.   2 marks

IMPORTANT INFORMATION

The couple should be referred to a clinical geneticist in case of an abnormal karyotype.

Products of conception should be collected in a sterile container with saline for karyotyping.

4. A 15-years-old girl admits to being sexually active. She wishes to use the combined oral contraceptive pills as she has heard a lot about them.

a. Highlight the relevant information that you will gather at this consultation.

(7 marks)

Note: This stem has 2 key issues. The woman is below the legal age of consent and the counselling deals with the first prescription of combined pills.

Identify the reason for this visit. Is she in a mutually agreeable relationship?

1 mark

Ask about the menstrual history and LMP. Assess need for emergency contraception. 1 mark

Assess her competence according to the Fraser guidelines. 1 mark

Review any possible contraindications in medical/drug/sexual or family history.

1 mark

Identify any factors amenable to use of combined contraceptive pills- menorrhagia, dysmennorhoea, irregular cycles, or acne vulgaris. 1 mark

Check her blood pressure, BMI and examine her breasts. 1 mark

Assess any additional counseling or support needs by her educational status, social and financial support. (Is she a drug addict? Or a child abuse victim?) 1 mark

b. Discuss the important side effects of OCP's that she needs to know?

(5 marks)

Pills are potentially very safe at her age and benefits outweigh side effects. If taken consistently and correctly, they are 99 percent safe in preventing pregnancy.

1 mark

Minor side effects are common in the first three months of use. These include breakthrough bleeding, nausea, breast tenderness, acne and a slight decrease in libido, most of which resolve with time. 2 marks

A slight increase in risk of heart attacks, strokes and blood clots is primarily seen in older or high-risk women. 1 mark

Certain medications, like antiepileptics may reduce their effectiveness and require additional contraceptive precautions during their use. 1 mark

**c. She decides to use the OCP's. Discuss the advice that you will give her.
(8 marks)**

She can start taking the pill anywhere from the first to the fifth day of her cycle. She needs to use additional protection either as abstinence or barriers for the first seven days. 2 marks

One pill has to be taken every day for 21 consecutive days, preferably at the same time of the day followed by a seven days gap. This will regularize her periods and reduce bleeding. 1 mark

Adequate advice on missed pills should be given. 1 mark

She will need additional protection during episodes of diarrhea, vomiting within 2 hours of pill intake or while on certain medications. She should inform her GP of pill use before taking any prescriptions. 1 mark

Encourage her to use the pill for at least three months before giving it up for any reason. She should come back for advice in case of any concerns like irregular bleeding or any untoward symptoms. 1 mark

Use of barriers and safe sex practises should be recommended at all times. The usefulness of taking a vaccine against HPV may be discussed. 1 mark

Encourage her to have proper nutrition, exercise and if applicable reduce her smoking. 1 mark

Time allowed: 1.45 hours   *MM 80*

1. A second gravida attends your clinic at 36 weeks gestation to discuss the pros and cons of her delivery. Her first delivery was by caesarean section for a breech presentation and she is medically fit.   **(7, 13 marks)**
    a. Which factors in her history will favour an elective repeat section?
    b. Write the issues of your counseling session as she wishes to undertake a trial for the VBAC.

2. An apparently healthy woman of Asian origin residing in UK wishes to travel to India for vacation. She is currently 24 weeks pregnant.
                                                                  (12, 4, 4 marks)
    a. Outline the general advice that you will give her.
    b. What are the contraindications to air travel in pregnancy?
    c. What specific vaccinations would she require before the travel?

3. a. Describe the common chemotherapeutic agents used in gynaecology and their side effects.   **(12, 8 marks)**
    b. What is chemoradiation? How does it help in treatment of gynaecological malignancies?

4. A 32-years-old woman was found to have bilateral endometriotic cysts on ultrasound. She has been trying to conceive for the last two years.
                                                                  (14, 6 marks)
    a. Discuss the relevant issues.
    b. She also has bilateral cornual block and wishes to conceive as soon as possible. What advice will you give to her?

1. **A second gravida attends your clinic at 36 weeks gestation to discuss the pros and cons of her delivery. Her first delivery was by caesarean section for a breech presentation and she is medically fit.**

a. **Which factors in her history will favour an elective repeat section?**
(7 marks)

Pregnant women with a previous section may be offered either planned VBAC (vaginal birth after C-section) or ERCS (Elective repeat C-section). New evidence is emerging to indicate that VBAC may not be as safe as originally thought. 1 mark

Body mass index more than 30 decreases the chances of a vaginal birth. 1 mark

Previous history and operative notes should be reviewed and history of a classical section scar or uterine incision other than the uncomplicated low transverse incision (T or J incision). The chances of a successful VBAC decrease if there has been an induced labour in the last pregnancy. 2 marks

If maternal preferences and priorities clearly lie in favour of a repeat caesarean section, she should be offered the same. 1 mark

Planned TOLAC (Trial of labor after C-section) is contraindicated if she is at high-risk of complications (history of extensive transfundal uterine surgery) or when vaginal delivery is contraindicated (noncephalic presentation, macrosomia or placenta praevia). 2 marks

b. **Write the issues of your counselling session as she wishes to undertake a trial for the VBAC.**
(13 marks)

The decision about mode of birth requires a thorough counselling of risks and benefits of a repeat section versus a vaginal delivery, shared patient- doctor decision making and importance of maternal preferences and priorities. Specific reasons for her request should be explored, discussed and recorded. 2 marks

The success rates for vaginal birth after caesarean section vary from 72 to 76 percent. 1 mark

With a repeat section there is decreased perineal pain, urinary incontinence (after 3 months) and uterovaginal prolapse. Risk of intrapartum infant death and neonatal morbidity is decreased in planned C-section. 3 marks

A VBAC avoids major abdominal surgery, lowers a women's risk of haemorrhage and infection and shortens the postpartum recovery. It may also help women avoid the possible future risks of having multiple caesareans and associated surgeries like hysterectomy, bladder and bowel injury, infections and abnormal placental conditions(praevia and accreta). 3 marks

Uterine rupture is a rare complication but the risk of dehiscence is higher with VBAC.   1 mark

Once a caesarean section, always a hospital delivery and there is no place for domiciliary management of such pregnancies.   1 mark

Details of the antenatal counselling should be documented in her notes. 1 mark

She should be provided with information leaflets.   1 mark

IMPORTANT INFORMATION

There is an increased incidence of abdominal pain, bladder and ureteric injury, need for further surgery (laparotomy, dilatation and curettage or hysterectomy), admission to intensive care unit, thromboembolic disease, longer hospital stay hospital readmissions and maternal death with a repeat section. If performed before 38 completed weeks, it can increase neonatal respiratory morbidity (transient tachypnea of the newborn). The implications for future pregnancies include an increased incidence of having no more children, placenta praevia, and morbidly adherent placenta, uterine rupture before labour and antepartum still birth.

Misoprostol should be avoided for labor induction/ augmentation in all CS cases.

2. **An apparently healthy woman of Asian origin residing in UK wishes to travel to India for vacation. She is currently 24 weeks pregnant.**

a. **Outline the general advice that you will give her.** (12 marks)

Journey from UK to India is a long haul flight ($\geq$ 4 hours duration). Reassure her that in the absence of major obstetrical or medical complications, air travel during pregnancy is quite safe. She should carry her case notes with her. 2 marks

She should take an overseas medical insurance policy to cover her prenatal check-ups or any other accidental medical expenses. 1 mark

Return flight restrictions should be checked with the individual airlines as most flights do not allow more than 34 weeks pregnant woman on board. Some airlines require a doctor's letter to confirm fitness to travel. 1 mark

Required vaccines and antimalarial prevention need to be taken before travel. She should wear long sleeved dresses and carry insect repellents with her. Chloroquine 300 mg weekly to be started one week before travel and continued till 4 weeks on return. 2 marks

Airport security devices and X-ray checks are safe during pregnancy. 1 mark

Aisle seat is preferable as can take frequent small walks inside the airline. She should take plenty of nonalcoholic beverages on board, maintain lower limb mobility and do deep breathing exercises to reduce the incidence of thromboembolism. TED stocking should be worn at all time during her flight. 2 marks

General food and water safety precautions should be taken care of at all times(Avoid raw meat, poultry and dairy products and drink safe water). Frequent small meals and avoiding tea, coffee and colas can help her to overcome jet lag early. 2 marks

Provide her with RCOG published patient information leaflet- "Travelling in pregnancy". 1 mark

b. **What are the contraindications to air travel in pregnancy?** (4 marks)

Women with Placenta praevia, sickle cell disease, severe hypertension and severe anemia (Hb less than 8.5 g %) should be advised against air travel. 2 marks

Women having previous history of preterm labor, placental abruption, multiple pregnancies, recent bleeding or any invasive procedure during 2 weeks prior to travel should be informed clearly about unexpected obstetrical emergencies and lack of medical facilities on board. 2 marks

c. Which specific vaccinations would she require before the travel?

(4 marks)

Vaccines recommended for travel to India are hepatitis A, polio (injectable instead of oral vaccine), tetanus toxoid, typhoid and tuberculosis (BCG). All pregnant women should be encouraged to take swine flu vaccine.   3 marks

Optional vaccines are meningococcal meningitis (Delhi, Nepal, Pakistan) and post exposure rabies vaccine (if required).   1mark

IMPORTANT INFORMATION

Women at high-risk of thromboembolism (obese, thrombophilia, SLE, etc) should be started on low dose aspirin three days before and on the day of journey. Alternatively LMWH (dalteparin- 5000 IU) single dose on the day of travel and one day after should suffice to counter the higher risk of thrombosis.

Vaccine Categories

1. *Live attenuated viruses: MMR, polio (OPV-Sabin), yellow fever, varicella – all are absolutely contraindicated in pregnancy except yellow fever which is permitted on travel to endemic areas.*
2. *Live attenuated bacteria: Tularemia, and BCG. Tularemia may be required in rabbit handlers and laboratory workers. Monteux test and BCG is contraindicated in pregnancy.*
3. *Killed viruses: Hepatitis B, influenza, rabies, polio (Salk).*
4. *Killed bacteria: Cholera, meningococcus, pneumococcus, typhoid, plague and pertussis.*
5. *Toxoids: Anthrax, tetanus-diphtheria.*
6. *Immunoglobulins: Can be used freely if required.*
   - *Hepatitis A and measles- prepared from pooled human serums*
   - *Botulism and diphtheria- prepared from horse serum*
   - *Hepatitis B, rabies, tetanus, varicella-hyperimmune.*

Vaccines that can be freely used in pregnancy are: Tetanus, rabies (post-exposure prophylaxis), influenza, pneumococcus, and hepatitis B.

Foetus may get passive immunity against neonatal Tetanus and influenza if mother was immunized during pregnancy.

Immunoglobulins should be used in pregnancy:
1. *After exposure to – measles, hep A, B, tetanus, chicken pox or rabies.*
2. *VZIG for newborns of mothers who develop chicken pox 5 days before, until 2 days after delivery.*
3. *All women without a history of chicken pox should be passively immunized with VZIG within 96 hours of an exposure to chicken pox.*

CDC web site can be checked for information on vaccines.

3. a. Describe the common chemotherapeutic agents used in gynaecology and their side-effects. **(12 marks)**

Chemotherapeutic agents are classified according to the cell phase they act upon and inhibit.

S phase (DNA synthesis) agents are alkylating agents like cyclophosphamide-haemorrhagic cystitis and leukemia, chlorambusil, melphalan- leukemia, ifosphamide – coma. 3 marks

Antitumour antibiotics like actinomycin D, doxorubicincardiotoxic and bleomycin -pulmonary fibrosis. 2 marks

Antimetabolites like 5-FU- cerebellar ataxia, and methotrexate- bone marrow toxicity. 2 marks

Platinum compounds like cisplatin- renal toxicity, deafness, and carboplatin-myelosuppression. 2 marks

Topoisomerase 11 inhibitors like etoposide have nonspecific side effects. **M phase agents** are vinca alkaloids like vinblastine-bone marrow toxicity, vincristine-neurotoxicity and paclitaxel- pulmonary fibrosis and arrhythmias. 3 marks

b. What is chemoradiation? How does it help in treatment of gynaecological malignancies? **(8 marks)**

It is a new modality of treatment primarily used for cervical cancer. Few chemotherapeutic agents when given concurrently with radiotherapy make the tumour cells more responsive to treatment. 2 marks

Commonly used radiation sensitizers are 5- Fluorouracil, cisplatin, mitomycin and hydroxyurea. 2 marks

It helps by synchronization of cell cycle, decreases the risk of cross resistance, and decreases the oxygen depleted fractions in the tumour tissue. 1 mark

It has the advantage of being used as neoadjuvant (before radiation) treatment or concurrent or postradiation adjuvant therapy. 2 marks

Chemoradiation has reduced the risk of disease recurrence in advanced stage cervical cancer by approximately 30 percent. 1 mark

4. A 32-years-old woman was found to have bilateral endometriotic cysts on ultrasound. She has been trying to conceive for the last two years.

a. Discuss the relevant issues. **(14 marks)**

Her concerns in terms of pain or infertility need to be prioritized.   2 marks

Medical management has no role in infertility due to endometriosis. Choice of medical management depends on several factors including previous treatment, severity of symptoms, and size of cysts and grade of endometriosis.   2 marks

Laparoscopic ablation of disease deposits along with bilateral cystectomy, instead of drainage and fulguration results in higher pregnancy rates. Tubal flushing increases her chances of conception.   2marks

Possibility of adjacent organ injury due to adhesions and possible laparotomy should be explained and written consent taken accordingly.   2 marks

Tubal patency, ovulation and sperm count need to be checked prior to any surgical intervention.   1 mark

General advice for smoking cessation, rubella immunity, cervical screening and preconceptional folic acid should be emphasized.   2 marks

Use of GnRH agonists 3 to 6 months before surgery may be considered for big and dense deposits. It also increases her chances before IVF.   2 marks

Assisted reproductive techniques should be started in the very next cycle after surgery.   1 mark

b. She also has bilateral cornual block and wishes to conceive as soon as possible. What advice will you give to her? **(6 marks)**

Assisted reproductive techniques offer her a better prognosis instead of tubal reconstruction.   2 marks

She should be referred to a specialist centre for *in vitro* fertilization.   1 mark

Laparoscopic ovarian cystectomy prior to IVF will improve her chances of conception.   2 marks

Inform her of the support groups and provide her with information leaflets.   1 mark

Time allowed: 1.45 hours   *MM 80*

1. You are the Registrar on duty and have admitted a primigravida, with term pregnancy, breech presentation and multiple fibroids for elective LSCS.   (7, 9, 4 marks)
   a. Enumerate your pre-operative checklist.
   b. What precautions will you take while performing her caesarean section?
   c. Describe her post-operative assessment.

2. A 37-year-old barrister has conceived following IVF treatment. She is currently seven weeks pregnant and an ultrasound scan reveals a gestational sac in the right fallopian tube.   (9, 11 marks)
   a. What are the issues you would counsel her about?
   b. Her serum β-HCG value is 3,700 IU, no cardiac activity is appreciable at present and she prefers to try the medical management. Describe your plan of management for her.

3. A 19-year-old woman with migraine requests long acting reversible contraceptives (LARC).   (4, 16 marks)
   a. What are the options for LARC?
   b. Describe the general and specific advantages and disadvantages of each method.

4. A couple presents to your clinic three years after marriage with primary infertility. The partner's semen analysis shows azoospermia.
   a. How will you investigate and manage him?   (15, 5 marks)
   b. He is found to have bilateral absence of vas deferens. He is keen to have a child of his own genetic material. What would you advise him?

1. **You are the Registrar on duty and have admitted a primigravida, with term pregnancy, breech presentation and multiple fibroids for elective LSCS.**

a. **Enumerate your pre-operative checklist.** **(7 marks)**

Explain to her the risks (blood loss, infection, thrombosis) and benefits of surgery. Check consent forms and explain about the surgery and aftercare.   2 marks

Repeat her fresh FBC and arrange blood according to Hb. If good Hb—group and save, otherwise have adequate blood in hand before surgery. Check Rhesus factor—if Rh negative—she will require appropriate doses of Anti-D.   2 marks

Recheck foetal presentation, placentation and number, size, position of fibroids on a fresh scan. Discuss the probable skin incision with her transverse or vertical midline, depending on the findings.   2 marks

Inform the relevant personnel about the time of surgery: these are the Ob/Gyn consultant, anaesthetist, haematologist, ODA, and concerned midwife. Speak to her partner as well.   1 mark

b. **What precautions will you take while performing her caesarean section?** **(9 marks)**

Perform the surgery under consultant supervision.   1 mark

Choose the skin incision according to scan findings.   1 mark

Uterine incision should be lower segment transverse if there is enough accessibility of lower uterine segment. May have to resort to upper segment classical section if big cervical/lower segment fibroids present.   2 marks

Delivery of the baby may be by Simple Breech extraction. Always identify the foot of the baby by the heel before taking it out. If difficulty is encountered in delivering the baby's head, forceps may be applied to the after-coming head; alternatively the incision may be converted to an inverted T-incision.   1 mark

Start uterotonics (oxytocin infusion), antibiotics and thromboprophylaxis after the delivery of baby.   2 marks

Uterine closure is in two layers for transverse incision and in three layers for upper segment sections. Ensure meticulous haemostasis. Upper segment is likely to ooze and an abdominal drain may be required.   1 mark

Skin closure will be by subcuticular sutures in transverse skin incision and single layer closure for vertical incisions.   1 mark

c. Describe her post-operative assessment. **(4 marks)**

In the immediate post-operative period assess her need for IV fluids, antibiotics, pain relief and thromboprophylaxis. Check vaginal bleeding and vital signs.

1 mark

Encourage breastfeeding and early ambulation. Indwelling urinary catheter should be removed according to the extent of lower segment dissection. 1 mark

Before discharge discuss contraception, lactation, cervical screening (if due) and follow-up postnatal visits. She may be able to have a normal vaginal delivery the next time if presentation and placentation are normal. Discuss the importance of follow-up scans to monitor her fibroids. Provide information leaflets if required.

2 marks

2. **A 37-year-old barrister has conceived following IVF treatment. She is currently seven weeks pregnant and an ultrasound scan reveals a gestational sac in the right fallopian tube.**

a. **What are the issues you would counsel her about?** (9 marks)

An ectopic pregnancy after an IVF cycle is emotionally a very traumatic event and the couple should be handled sympathetically. At the same time we have to be legally right so meticulous documentation and case notes of the counselling session should be kept. 1 mark

During embryo transfer, even if embryos are replaced in the uterine cavity under ultrasound guidance, there may be retrograde migration resulting in a tubal pregnancy. In UK, 11 per 1000 pregnancies are ectopics and the incidence is much higher in IVF pregnancies. 1 mark

This pregnancy is not growing at the right place and is not viable. There is no known method to bring it into the uterus and we quickly have to stop its growth otherwise it may rupture and cause excessive bleeding inside thereby endangering the mother's life. 2 marks

The choice of treatment can be surgical or with drugs. Expectant management has no role because of high incidence of tubal rupture and internal bleeding. 1 mark

Surgical approach is by laparoscopy as long as she is haemodynamically stable. If the left tube is normal, looks healthy, we prefer to remove the whole of right tube (salpingectomy) along with the contents of pregnancy. 1 mark

If she had IVF for tubal factor this time, chances are that both her tubes are damaged. Consent may be taken for a bilateral salpingectomy to reduce her chances of a repeat ectopic. 1 mark

Medical management is by single intramuscular injection of methotrexate. She will have to come often to the hospital for follow-up and may still require a surgical intervention. 1 mark

Explain to her that tubes have no role in an IVF pregnancy and she may conceive again with help and have an intrauterine healthy pregnancy the next time. Allow her as many counselling sessions as she requires. 1 mark

b. **Her serum β-HCG value is 3,700 IU, no cardiac activity is appreciable at present and she prefers to try the medical management. Describe your plan of management for her.** (11 marks)

With β-HCG value around 3000, no cardiac activity and haemodynamic stability, she is a good candidate for medical management with methotrexate therapy. It would be as effective as the surgical treatment for her. 2 marks

Single dose methotrexate is given by intramuscular injection in a dose of 50 mg/ m^2 of body surface area on day 1. 1 mark

Provide her with information leaflets informing her about further treatment and adverse effects of the drug. Three out of four patients will have some abdominal pain on treatment. She may require hospitalisation for observation if it is severe.
2 marks

Some women experience conjunctivitis, mouth ulcers and stomach upsets during treatment. Seven per cent women may have tubal rupture and one in ten women requires surgical intervention after methotrexate therapy. 1 mark

250 IU of anti D should be administered if she is rhesus negative. 1 mark

She is asked to return on day 4 and 7 for her β-HCG test. If these two readings show a decline of less than 15 per cent, give her an additional dose of methotrexate injection. Fifteen per cent of all women undergoing treatment may require an additional dose. 1 mark

Surgical intervention may be required if there are symptoms of intra-abdominal bleeding. 1 mark

Arrange adequate follow-up and provide her with the hospital emergency contact number so she can return anytime. Inform her GP. 1 mark

She should be asked to avoid sexual intercourse during treatment, maintain adequate fluid intake and avoid pregnancy for the next three months. 1 mark

3. A 19-year-old woman with migraine requests long acting reversible contraceptives (LARC).

a. What are the options for LARC? **4 marks**

The recommended LARCs are the copper intrauterine devices, progestogen only intrauterine systems, progestogen only injectable contraceptives, and progestogen only subdermal implants. 4 marks

b. Describe the general and specific advantages and disadvantages of each method. **(4, 12 marks)**

The biggest advantage of LARC is that its effectiveness is not dependent on daily concordance by the user. All currently available LARC methods are more cost-effective than the combined pill even at 1 year of use. These are quite effective in preventing unwanted pregnancy. 3 marks

Copper intrauterine devices have a long and reversible contraceptive life of 5 to 10 years depending on the amount of copper. There is no delay in return of fertility after removal. It does not affect the body weight and can be safely used by breastfeeding women, diabetic and even HIV positive women. 2 marks

Intrauterine devices may cause pain and unacceptable vaginal bleeding (almost 50% women discontinue its use within 5 years). 1 mark

There is a small procedure related risk of uterine perforation (1 in 1000), pelvic infections (1 in 100), expulsions (1 in 20 women in 5 years) and failure of contraception leading to pregnancy (less than 20 in 1000 in 5 years). 2 marks

Progestogen intrauterine system (IUS- Mirena) provides good contraception till 5 years (failure rate of 10 in 1000 over 5 years), causes no weight gain and is good for women with menorrhagia, migraine, venous thromboembolism and other estrogen dependent conditions. 2 marks

IUS may cause irregular bleeding, spotting and pain in the first-six months of insertion (60% women discontinue its use within 5 years), and increases the likelihood of developing acne. There is a very small-risk of uterine perforation (1 in 1000), pelvic infection (1 in 100) and expulsion (1 in 20 women in 5 years). 2 marks

Progestogen only injectable contraceptives are safe for women with migraines, oestrogen dependent conditions and may reduce the frequency of seizures in epileptic women. 1 mark

These may cause an increase in weight (2-3 kg in 1 year), altered bleeding pattern and amenorrhoea (50% stop its use within 1 year), a small loss in bone mineral density and a delay of up to one year for return of fertility after stopping its use. 1 mark

Progestogen only subdermal implants (implanon) prevents pregnancy for 3 years (failure rates of 1 in 1000 in 3 years), does not delay return of fertility on removal, reduces dysmenorrhoea, and is not associated with changes in weight, mood, libido or headache. 1 mark

It has the disadvantage of flaring acne and causing irregular bleeding pattern which may last throughout. 1 mark

IMPORTANT NOTE

Long acting reversible methods of contraception (LARCs) require administration less than once every cycle or month. At present LARC usage is around 8 to 10 per cent in UK in 19 to 49 age group. Combined vaginal rings are not yet approved by the UK marketing agencies (till 2005) for LARC.

Intrauterine devices (IUD), intrauterine system (IUS) and implants are more cost-effective than the injectable contraceptives.

Risk of ectopic pregnancy is lower in women with IUD and IUS than when using no contraception.

Progestogen only injectable contraceptives have a low failure rate (4 in 1000 over 2 years). Pregnancy rates with the use of depo-medroxyprogesterone acetate (DMPA) are lower than with norethisterone acetate (NET-EN). DMPA needs to be given every 12 weeks and NET-EN every 8 weeks. Amenorrhoea is more likely with DMPA, is not harmful and the incidence increases with repeated injections. Women with amenorrhoea on DMPA still need to use an alternative contraception, if amenorrhoea persists after discontinuation of injectables.

4. A couple present to your clinic three years after marriage with primary infertility. The partner's semen analysis shows azoospermia.

a. How will you investigate and manage him?   **(15 marks)**

A single semen sample is not sufficient to label the man as azoospermic and should be repeated on at least two other occasions at least two weeks apart. The cycle of spermatogenesis is 12 weeks long and any systemic illness/insult 3 months ago may produce transient azoospermia.   2 marks

The presence of fructose in the semen will confirm the patency of the vas deferens while its absence will suggest obstructive azoospermia.   2 marks

History of smoking, intake of drugs especially marijuana and alcohol should be elicited. Sexual history and possibility of anorgasm or retrograde ejaculation should be kept in mind. To confirm the diagnosis, the bladder should be emptied and postorgasmic urine sample should be centrifuged to look for spermatozoa.   2 marks

Clinical examination should be performed to see the presence and size of the testicles.

If the testicles are normal in size, the vas deferens should be palpated bilaterally. If the testicles are undescended, a surgical opinion should be sought. If the testicles are small and atrophic, this may be a case of primary testicular failure which can be confirmed on fine needle aspiration cytology (FNAC).   2 marks

Hormonal evaluation should include FSH/LH/testosterone and prolactin. If testosterone levels are low, testosterone therapy should be initiated. If FSH and LH levels are low indicating hypogonadotropic hypogonadism, therapy should be commenced with weekly injections of HCG and should be continued for at least 12 weeks. If prolactin levels are high, destress programmes and bromocriptine therapy should be initiated. Any therapy commenced will show result after three months.   3 marks

In complete productive azoospermia, levels of FSH and LH will be raised, testicles will be atrophic and FNAC will show no spermatogonia. Here treatment options will involve donor semen.   2 marks

In partial productive azoospermia, FNAC will show some spermatogenesis. If spermatids are visible, the option of testicular sperm aspiration and ICSI should be offered with a caution that success rates are only 23 to 30 per cent per cycle. If spermatids are not produced, round cell sperm Injection or ROSI can be performed. However, the pregnancy rates are lower 15 to 20 per cent.   2 marks

b. He is found to have bilateral absence of vas deferens. He is keen to have a child with his own genetic material. What would you advise him?

(5 marks)

It is a congenital condition and at present it is not possible to implant the vas deferens surgically. 1 mark

It is possible to harvest good sperms from the epididymis by percutaneous sperm aspiration (PESA) and then proceeding with IVF-ICSI. Pregnancy rates of over 30 per cent have been achieved in good assisted reproductive techniques (ART) centres. 2 marks

However, the possibility of propagating the same disorder in the male offspring exists and the couple should be referred to a genetic clinic for counselling.

1 mark

The female partner should have her complete workup including the tubal patency tests and follicular monitoring prior to initiating any ART procedures. 1 mark

1. A 30-year-old woman has recently been diagnosed as having Systemic Lupus Erythematosis (SLE). She wishes to start her family and comes to you for advice.   (8, 12 marks)
   a. Briefly outline her pre-conception counselling.
   b. How will you manage her prenatal period?

2. You are the Obstetrics and Gynaecology Senior Registrar (Specialist Registrar Year 3) in a unit delivering 4,500 women per year. It is mid-afternoon, and suddenly the emergency buzzer goes off in Room 6 and an anxious midwife puts her head out of the door and shouts "patient haemorrhaging".   (10, 10 marks)
   a. Describe your immediate actions and the personnel you would liaison with.
   b. The midwife informs you that her pulse is 120 per minute, blood pressure 100/70 mmHg and she is getting restless. Her placenta has been removed completely and you assess her visual blood loss to be around 750 ml. Describe your further course of actions.

3. A 15-year-old woman presents with primary amenorrhoea and cyclical pain. Her hormonal profile is normal and she has normal secondary sexual characters.   (7, 6, 7 marks)
   a. What history and examination will you do to reach a diagnosis?
   b. Discuss the differential diagnosis.
   c. What additional investigations will you undertake to reach a diagnosis and what are your principles of management.

4. A 25-year-old with 8 weeks amenorrhoea is diagnosed as complete molar pregnancy on ultrasound.   (14, 6 marks)
   a. Describe your clinical management of the patient including counselling.
   b. Four months later she comes with persistent bleeding. What additional investigations will you consider and outline your principles of management at this time.

1. **A 30-year-old woman has recently been diagnosed as having Systemic Lupus Erythematosis (SLE). She wishes to start her family and comes to you for advice.**

a. **Briefly outline her pre-conception counselling.** (8 marks)

SLE is a systemic connective tissue disease characterised by periods of disease activity (flares) and remissions. Severe disease flare may be potentially life-threatening and foetomaternal outcome is improved if disease is in remission for at least 6 months prior to conception. 1 mark

Knowledge of the antiphospholipid, anti-Ro, anti-La antibody, renal and blood pressure status and immunosuppressive therapy allows prediction of the risks to the women and her foetus. Six per cent women have associated autoimmune disorders and appropriate investigations should be advised for the same. 2 marks

Some drug therapies are teratogenic and foetotoxic. Appropriate dose adjustments to achieve optimal control should be established. If possible, discontinue methotrexate, mycophenolate and cyclophosphamide for at least three months prior to conception due to long half-life and possible teratogenicity. 2 marks

Counsel her regarding increased potential for SLE flares, spontaneous miscarriage, intrauterine growth restriction during pregnancy, pre-eclampsia, preterm delivery and foetal death. In the absence of renal disease the pregnancy outcome is similar to that of general population. 1 mark

Prescribe effective contraception till medical optimisation is achieved. 1 mark

Check her rubella status, cervical screening, folic acid supplementation and advise her to avoid smoking. 1 mark

b. **How will you manage her antenatal period?** (12 marks)

Antenatal care should be undertaken by a multidisciplinary team, in a tertiary care setting with experienced staff. 1 mark

Encourage early booking with a first trimester scan to establish accurate dates. Maintain antenatal schedule of 2 weeks till the second trimester and weekly thereafter. 1 mark

Baseline investigations include full blood counts (anaemia and thrombocytopaenia), renal functions, double stranded DNA (ds DNA), anti-Ro, La, Smith and anticardiolipin antibodies and lupus anticoagulant, urinalysis for proteinuria and red cell casts. If she has known renal disease, 24 hours urinary proteins and creatinine clearance should be done. Repeat appropriate investigations at 4 weekly intervals. 2 marks

Watch for signs and symptoms of SLE flare. These include hypertension, haematuria with rising proteinuria and red cell casts on urinalysis. Investigation shows increasing titres of ds DNA, serum creatinine, normal C-reactive protein (CRP) and falling complement levels (C3, C4) with thrombocytopaenia.   1 mark

Foetal surveillance with regular growth scans after 20 weeks, Doppler velocimetry at 24 weeks and regularly thereafter, to detect foetal growth restriction at the earliest should be undertaken. If mother has positive anti-Ro, anti-La antibodies, foetal echocardiography should be done at 22 weeks to detect congenital heart block in foetus. Fetal P-R interval measurements, if available can detect first degree heart block.   2 marks

Low-dose aspirin therapy and LMWH (low molecular weight heparin) should be considered if antiphospholipid antibodies are positive. Dexamethasone, salbutamol or digoxin therapy may be judiciously used to convert second degree heart blocks to first and if hydrops foetalis develops.   2 marks

Glucocorticoids (Prednisolone) can be safely used during pregnancy and to manage flares. Nonsteroidal anti inflammatory drugs (NSAIDs) particularly Cox -2 selective inhibitors, should be avoided after second trimester. Azathioprine and hydroxychloroquine are the second line therapy and may be continued throughout pregnancy. Methotrexate and cyclosporin are third line therapy. Severe flares may require pulsed methyl prednisolone therapy. Avoid antimalarials and full dose NSAIDs. Hypertension is controlled with nifedipine or hydralazine.   2 marks

Deliver at term in absence of complications; avoid postdates. Notify pediatrician and anaesthetist at the time of delivery. Steroid boluses may be required at delivery for patients on chronic steroid therapy. The risk of neonatal lupus is increased if a previous child has been affected but is not related to the severity of maternal disease.   1 mark

2. **You are the Obstetrics and Gynaecology Senior Registrar (Specialist Registrar Year 3) in a unit delivering 4,500 women per year. It is mid-afternoon, and suddenly the emergency buzzer goes off in Room 6 and an anxious midwife puts her head out of the door and shouts "patient haemorrhaging".**

a. **Describe your immediate actions and the personnel you would liaison with.** **(10 marks)**

Note: The practical management of PPH may be considered as having at least four components: **communication**; with all relevant professionals; **resuscitation**; **monitoring** and **investigations**.

Minor blood loss without any clinical signs of shock require basic measures of monitoring and 'readiness for resuscitation', whereas an estimated loss of more than 1000 ml (or a smaller loss associated with clinical signs of shock, tachycardia, hypotension, tachypnoea, oliguria or delayed peripheral capillary filling) prompts a full protocol of measures to resuscitate, monitor and arrest the bleeding.

Go to room 6, quickly find out the patient's name and rapidly introduce yourself in a calm confident manner. 1 mark

Ask someone at the reception desk/nurses station to put out an emergency call to the duty Anaesthetic Registrar, Operating Department Assistant (ODA), and obstetric SHO if not present. Ask Obstetric Nursing Officer to arrange extra staff and the most easily available experienced midwife for room 6. The person concerned will then inform blood bank technician and haematologist about the situation along with the details of the patient. Porters should be summoned to maternity unit for carrying the samples. Her partner should also be apprised of the situation. 2 marks

Consultant haematologist and obstetrician should be informed of the clinical situation. Theatre should be informed for a possible intervention. 1 mark

Put a hand on the mother's abdomen to palpate the uterus and ascertain its tone and size, whilst simultaneously "rubbing up" a contraction. 1 mark

Ask the staff midwife for baseline vitals, i.e. pulse, BP and a rapid summary of what has happened so far, including whether or not the placenta is delivered and is complete or not. Make a visual impression about the estimated blood loss.
1 mark

Make an assessment of the mother's cardiovascular state, particularly her pulse rate, and lower the upper part of her bed so that she is lying horizontally. Assign one nurse solely for record keeping; patient's vital signs, urine output, amount and type of all fluids the patient receives, dosage and type of drugs given.   1 mark

Insert two large size intravenous cannulae, (preferably 14 gauge) and take 20 ml blood samples from the mother for full blood count, clotting studies and cross matching, and order at least 6 units of blood. Connect an infusion of Haemaccel solution in one and Hartmann's solution in the other line.   1 mark

Give the mother oxygen to breathe via a face mask, and put a warming blanket over mother's abdomen. Ask the staff midwife to insert a Foley catheter into the mother's bladder and connect to a drainage bag. Give the mother an intramuscular injection of syntometrine if not hypertensive.   1 mark

If placenta and membranes are undelivered, make a further attempt at controlled cord traction and if unsuccessful, proceed to manual removal in theatre.   1 mark

b. **The midwife informs you that her pulse is 120 per minute, blood pressure 100/70 mmHg and she is getting restless. Her placenta has been removed completely and you assess her visual blood loss to be around 750 ml. Describe your further course of actions.   (10 marks)**

Visual blood loss estimation often underestimates the total loss. If bleeding still continues and uterus is relaxed, commence infusion with 10 units' syntocinon. $PGF_{2\alpha}$ (.5-1 mg) can be given straight into uterine muscle, provided she is not asthmatic. Examine the placenta for completeness. Give further bolus of oxytocin if required. Rule out rupture or inversion of uterus.   2 marks

Rule out trauma to vulva, vagina and cervix if uterus remains contracted and bleeding continues.   1 mark

If bleeding continues, she may need to be taken to theatre to explore the uterus for any retained products of conception, trauma or inversion. Apply bimanual compression till anaesthesia is administered. Four units of whole blood, 2 units' fresh frozen plasma and one unit factor VIII should be ready in the theatre.

2 marks

Exclude coagulation disorder by the preliminary results. Ensure that patient remains haemodynamically stable, replace lost blood, platelets and clotting factors. Keep PT/aPTT ratio to more than 1.5 times normal and consider CVP monitoring if large volumes of fluids and blood products are required to be administered.   1 mark

Uterine packing or balloon tamponade may be tried before shifting the patient to theatre for further exploration.   1 mark

Explain her condition and the possibility of embolisation/internal iliac ligation/ hysterectomy to the attendant.   1 mark

In the theatre, the following procedures should be tried in order—haemostatic brace sutures, bilateral uterine artery ligation, selective arterial embolisation and finally hysterectomy.   2 marks

IMPORTANT NOTE

The decision for hysterectomy should be taken sooner and at least two consultants should be involved in decision making.

3. A 15-year-old woman presents with primary amenorrhoea and cyclical pain. Her hormonal profile is normal and she has normal secondary sexual characters.

a. What history and examination will you undertake to reach a diagnosis? (7 marks)

History of regularity of cyclical pain at the same time each month should be elicited.
1 mark

Presence of secondary sexual characters, e.g. axillary and pubic hair as well as breast development should be confirmed.
2 marks

Local vulval examination with parting of the labia will confirm an imperforate hymen. Some cases may show a bulge in the hymenal area with bluish/black tinge due to collected blood.
2 marks

Ultrasound scan of the lower abdomen will confirm the presence of ovaries and uterus. There will be haematocolpos and in some chronic cases there may also be haematometra and/or haematosalpinx.
2 marks

b. Discuss the differential diagnosis. (6 marks)

The most likely diagnosis is cryptomenorrhoea due to an imperforate hymen or rarely due to cervical/vaginal stenosis.
2 marks

Differential diagnosis includes other causes of primary amenorrhoea with co-incidental abdominal pain due to gastrointestinal causes.
1 mark

Other causes of primary amenorrhoea are chromosomal aberrations like Turners Syndrome (XO), functional hypothalamic amenorrhoea due to excessive exercise, eating disorders like anorexia, physical or psychological stress.
2 marks

Osteogenesis imperfecta, pituitary tumors, lack of reproductive organs e.g. absent uterus in Mayer, Rokitansky syndrome, non- communicating horn of a bicornuate uterus, and transverse vaginal septum are other rare causes.
1 mark

c. What additional investigations will you undertake to reach a diagnosis and what are your principles of management. (7 marks)

In cases of abnormal development of reproductive organs, ultrasound should include visualisation of the kidneys and bladder to rule out congenital renal anomalies like horseshoe kidney, pelvic kidney, double ureter or unilateral renal agenesis. Occasionally haematocolpos can be associated with pressure effects on the kidneys resulting in hydronephrosis.
2 marks

MRI scan of the abdomen and pelvis along with ultrasound scan may be required to establish the status of the reproductive organs and kidneys.　　1 mark

Intravenous pyelogram will confirm the presence of double ureter which may be otherwise difficult to visualise. It will also provide information on whether the renal tissue in a horse-shoe kidney is functional or non-functional.　　1 mark

Management of cryptomenorrhoea consists of making a cruciate incision in the imperforate hymen under general anaesthesia and allowing complete drainage of collected blood. If there is concomitant presence of haematometra, cervical dilatation and drainage of the uterus should be performed.　　2 marks

Prophylactic broad spectrum antibiotic cover should be administered to prevent secondary bacterial infection.　　1 mark

4. A 25-year-old woman with 8 weeks amenorrhoea is diagnosed as complete molar pregnancy on ultrasound.

a. Describe your clinical management of the patient including counselling.
(14 marks)

Haematological investigations including baseline serum beta HCG, full blood count, blood group and cross matching, thyroid function tests, urea, electrolytes and liver function tests should be performed.   2 marks

She should also be investigated for distant metastasis which should include an X-ray chest and ultrasound of the abdomen.   1 mark

It should be explained that her pregnancy will need termination as there is no foetal development.   1 mark

Information leaflets should be provided and she should be put in contact with support groups.   1 mark

Consent should be obtained for suction evacuation under general anaesthesia, blood should be cross matched and anti-D should be administered in full dose if rhesus negative.   2 marks

During suction evacuation, concomitant use of uterotonic agents like oxytocin will reduce the amount of bleeding. Suction should be performed gently and sharp curettage should be avoided as it may lead to perforation.   2 marks

If complete evacuation is not possible in one sitting, repeat curettage can be performed after a week. Ultrasound guided evacuation will help to reduce the chances of incomplete evacuation. Removed products should be sent for histopathology and grading.   2 marks

Serum beta HCG should be monitored every week until it is negative and then she is followed-up by urinary levels. The length of follow-up depends on the rapidity of fall in serum values and is informed by the referral center by post.   1 mark

She should be advised to postpone pregnancy until her urinary HCG levels have been negative for one year. Oral contraceptive pills are safe after beta HCG has become negative. Double barrier protection should be advocated.   2 marks

b. Four months later she comes with persistent bleeding. What additional investigations will you consider and outline your principles of management at this time.   **(6 marks)**

Repeat registration and consultation with the screening centers at Sheffield, Dundee or Charing Cross should be sought before intervention.   1 mark

Persistent Gestational Trophoblastic Disease (GTD) occurs in 10 per cent of the women after a complete molar pregnancy. Serum beta HCG levels should be repeated.   1 mark

Ultrasound scan of whole abdomen should be performed to look for retained tissue and/or a pregnancy/invasive mole or metastasis in liver due to choriocarcinoma.   1 mark

Brain and or chest imaging with an X- ray or CT scan should be done to rule out lung and brain metastases.   1 mark

Treatment will depend on the ultrasound findings and distant metastases. Multiple agent chemotherapy with methotrexate and folinic acid is required to treat invasive mole and choriocarcinoma. If there is no desire for future fertility, hysterectomy may be performed with the mole in situ. This can be followed by chemotherapy.
                                                                   2 marks

IMPORTANT NOTES

The incidence of GTN is 1 in 714 live births in UK. GTN includes hydatidiform mole, invasive mole, choriocarcinoma, and placental site tumour.

Complete moles are diploid (46, XX) with no foetal tissues and androgenetic in origin, i.e. no maternal tissues (consequence of duplication of haploid sperm or rarely a dispermic fertilisation of an empty ovum).

Partial moles are triploid (one set of maternal and 2 sets of paternal haploid genes) and have evidence of foetal tissues.

Time allowed: 1.45 hours   *MM 80*

1. A nulliparous woman presents at 34 weeks of pregnancy in the labour ward with rupture of membranes. Vaginal swab shows growth of group B Streptococcus.   **(15, 5 marks)**
   a. How does this information alter your management?
   b. Which factors would you look for in the history which may alert you to the possibility of the foetus getting infected with GBS.

2. A 35-year-old woman has been referred to you because her routine anomaly scan at 20 weeks has shown presence of solitary choroid plexus cyst.   **(14, 6 marks)**
   a. Highlight the major issues involved in counselling.
   b. Her elder sister, who is now 36 years old, had a baby affected by Down's syndrome last year. She wants to avoid the same fate for her pregnancy. How will you alley her fears?

3. A 24-year-old nulliparous woman complains of recurrent severe bloating sensation, difficulty in sleeping and breast tenderness. She appears irritable and reveals that her periods are due in about a week.   **(12, 8 marks)**
   a. Enumerate the management options available to her.
   b. What advice will you give to the patient as far as the symptom control is concerned?

4. A baby has just been delivered in the labour ward with ambiguous looking genitalia. Baby is otherwise normal. You are the registrar on duty.   **(6, 4, 10 marks)**
   a. What advice will you give the parents regarding the condition?
   b. Enumerate the differential diagnosis.
   c. How will you investigate and manage the baby?

1. **A nulliparous woman presents at 34 weeks of pregnancy in the labour ward with rupture of membranes. Vaginal swab shows growth of group B Streptococcus.**

a. **How does this information alter your management?** **(15 marks)**

Vaginal colonization with group B streptococcus (GBS) is associated with premature rupture of membranes and preterm delivery beyond 32 weeks. 2 marks

There are higher chances of intra-amniotic infections, postpartum endometritis, and puerperal septicemia. 1 mark

She should be offered admission in the hospital and standard labour ward protocol followed to administer tests of maternal and foetal well-being. 2 marks

Antenatal corticosteroids should be administered. 1 mark

A per vaginal examination, should be avoided if expectant management is contemplated. Daily white cell counts should be done and labour augmented if there is any sign of infection. A vaginal examination should be done prior to augmentation to check cervical dilatation and presenting part. 2 marks

Antibiotic chemoprophylaxis for GBS is not necessary unless she is in established labour. 1 mark

If labour is established or she has ≥ 2 risk factors, chemoprophylaxis should be administered as soon as possible after onset of labour and at least 2 hours before delivery. Recommended prophylaxis regimens are:

• Penicillin G 5 MU intravenously, followed by 2.5 MU IV every 4 hours, or

• Ampicillin 3 g IV followed by 1.5 g every 4 hours during labour or

• Clindamycin 900 mg IV every 8 hours. 2 marks

If chorioamnionitis is suspected broad spectrum antibiotic therapy including an agent active against GBS should replace GBS specific antibiotic prophylaxis.
1 mark

Pediatrician should be present to clinically evaluate the baby after birth. Close supervision must be maintained for at least 12 hours after delivery. If mother had ≥ 2 risk factors, blood cultures should be obtained and treatment initiated with Penicillin till culture results are available. 2 marks

Breastfeeding is not contraindicated. 1 mark

b. Which factors would you look for in the history which may alert you to the possibility of the foetus getting infected with GBS? (5 marks)

Delivery at <37 weeks, duration of rupture of membranes ≥18 hours, and intrapartum fever ≥ 38.0°C are risk factors for development of early onset (less than 7 days) neonatal GBS. 3 marks

If the mother had a previous baby affected by GBS, or GBS bacteriuria detected during the current pregnancy she is at a higher-risk of vaginal GBS colonisation during labour. Approximately 60 per cent of neonates with early onset disease had one or more of the above risk factors. 2 marks

IMPORTANT INFORMATION

GBS is facultative anaerobic gram-positive cocci and can be grown on non-selective media. However, optimal discovery rates require selective media. It can be recovered from vagina or cervix in up to 25 percent of pregnant women at some point during gestation. In majority it is innocuous to mother and baby but in 1/1000 deliveries it causes overwhelming neonatal infection which can be fatal or permanently disabling.

The incidence of early onset GBS in UK is 0.5/1000 live births. Mortality from GBS in term babies is 6 per cent and in preterm babies is 18 per cent.

In the USA, there is routine bacteriological screening for GBS of all pregnant patients between 35 to 37 weeks of pregnancy by means of vaginal and rectal swabs. All positive cases are given intrapartum antibiotic prophylaxis with ampicillin or intravenous penicillin.

UK does not recommend universal routine screening and treatment for GBS at present because of the potential risks of fatal anaphylaxis, the medicalisation of labour and the neonatal period, and infection with resistant organisms. The numbers of women that are required to be treated with antibiotics to prevent one neonatal death are very high and universal screening is not cost-effective for them.

UK guidelines do not recommend antenatal treatment of GBS even if discovered incidentally. However treatment during labour is effective in preventing morbidity and should be initiated, if GBS is discovered at that time.

2. **A 35-year-old woman has been referred to you because her routine anomaly scan at 20 weeks has shown presence of solitary choroid plexus cyst.**

a. **Highlight the major issues involved in counselling.** (14 marks)

Choroid Plexus (CP) cysts are found in approximately 1 per cent of routine second trimester scans. They are often transient and usually resolve between 22-26 weeks of gestation. As the only finding on ultrasound scan, these lack clinical significance.
3 marks

The couple should preferably be counselled together by a specialist and handled sympathetically in a quiet area specially dedicated for counselling. She should be seen within 24 hours of the scan within the same hospital or not more than two days later if referred.
2 marks

Choroids plexus cysts are considered 'Soft Markers' for foetal aneuploidy. These are usually transient ultrasound features which may indicate a risk of serious foetal chromosomal anomaly but which may in themselves be inconsequential.
2 marks

Five per cent such foetuses are associated with trisomy 18 and another 1 per cent have other karyotypic abnormalities. Presence of two or more markers increases the possibility of abnormal karyotype in foetus. Majority of affected foetuses have other structural abnormalities or dysmorphic features on ultrasound.
3 marks

Look for the presence of other soft markers (increased nuchal fold thickness, pyelectasis, hyperechogenic bowel, short femur, cardiac echogenic foci, etc.) including the subtle ones like overlapping fingers, micrognathia, club foot and sandal gap. Dandy walker malformation should be specifically looked for.
3 marks

Always offer a second opinion if demanded by the couple. Written information in the form of information leaflets should be provided to her.
1 mark

b. **Her elder sister who is now 36 years old, had a baby affected by Down's syndrome last year. She wants to avoid the same fate for her pregnancy. How will you alley her fears?** (6 marks)

Keeping her age in mind, offer amniocentesis to determine foetal karyotype, since the age related risk for trisomy 18 and 21 is higher than the accepted threshold for amniocentesis (1 in 274).
1 mark

0.5 per cent foetal loss associated with amniocentesis should be explained to her and she should be allowed to make an informed decision.
1 mark

Her risk of Down's syndrome however, remains the same with or without choroid plexus cysts. 2 marks

Offer termination of pregnancy if abnormal karyotype is found. If she decides to continue the pregnancy, offer to arrange a meeting with a pediatrician. 2 marks

IMPORTANT INFORMATION

Any women >31 years with isolated CP cysts should be offered amniocentesis. If she is younger, and there are no other ultrasound features, karyotyping is not required as the accumulated risks due to amniocentesis are higher.

Presence of single or multiple cysts or their subsequent disappearance do not alter the foetal prognosis.

3. **A 24-year-old nulliparous woman complains of recurrent severe bloating sensation, difficulty in sleeping and breast tenderness. She appears irritable and reveals that her periods are due in about a week.**

a. **Enumerate the management options available to her.** **(12 marks)**

Premenstrual syndrome (PMS) or Premenstrual dysphoric disorder (PMDD) is the most likely diagnosis. The management options are mainly symptomatic and have to be tailored to suit the patient's symptoms. 2 marks

PMS shows a strong placebo effect. She should be handled sympathetically, and the likely aetiology explained for reassurance. 2 marks

Lifestyle changes are likely to help. The use of surgery is not an option due to her young age. 1 mark

Evening primrose oil may be effective especially for relieving the breast symptoms. Supplements of vitamin B_6 (pyridoxine), vitamin E, and gamma linoleic acid have also shown to be of some value. 1 mark

Combined contraceptive pill preparations may be effective by suppressing ovulation. Ethinyl oestradiol and drospirenone containing pills have been found to be effective due to its antimineralocorticoid action. 1 mark

Danazol 100-200 mg daily is effective in treating breast symptoms but may cause unacceptable side effects like hirsutism. 1 mark

GnRH agonists like Triptorelin or Luprolide are of limited value as they are costly, may cause osteopenia and can only be used for short periods of 6 months.
1 mark

Severe bloating and weight gain may require the use of diuretics like Spironolactone, or Frusemide for short periods each month. NSAIDs may be added in the late luteal phase for any associated dysmenorrhea. 1 mark

Insomnia can be treated with anxiolytics like alprazolam or sedatives. Selective serotonin reuptake inhibitors like Fluoxitene 20 mg are becoming the first line therapy for PMDD because they are effective, well-tolerated and free of major side effects. In depressive mood disorders, tricyclic antidepressants have been used. 2 marks

b. **What advice will you give to the patient as far as the symptom control is concerned?** **(8 marks)**

Around 20 percent of women in reproductive age group suffer from PMS and she is not alone. 1 mark

Keeping a symptom diary and talking about the symptoms to a supportive person or group may help. 2 marks

General measures include exercising; 30 min a day, three times a week will help to elevate her mood by increasing endorphin levels.   1 mark

Relaxation techniques including meditation and yoga may be beneficial and reduce stress.   1 mark

Encourage her to eat a well-balanced diet with low salt and fat content to reduce premenstrual bloating. Taking vitamin B supplements may reduce her bloating and have an antidepressant effect.   1 mark

Adding bran to the diet will help in avoiding constipation which happens frequently during premenstrual period.   1 mark

Alcohol, chocolate, dairy products and caffeinated beverages may accentuate her irritability and their intake should be restricted.   1 mark

IMPORTANT NOTE

Three categories of symptoms have been recognised for PMDD:
- *Physical – headache, bloating, joint and muscle aches, breast tenderness and swelling*
- *Behavioral – poor concentration, insomnia, appetite changes, and social withdrawal*
- *Mood changes – depression, anxiety, irritability and mood swings.*

For the diagnosis the symptoms should have been present for at least four out of the previous six months. It is a diagnosis of exclusion and there are no laboratory tests for it. Diagnostic tools like COPE (calendar of premenstrual experiences) are used for follow-up.

Its management is important because the symptoms of PMDD can lead to socio-economic loss, and secondly because of associated legal implications that arise in conjunction with personal accountability in cases of PMDD.

Differential diagnosis include-Molimina, situational stress disorders and chronic affective disorders.

Molimina are the symptoms that women experience premenstrually. These are the same as PMS symptoms but are milder and allow a woman to carry on her normal activities.

Situational stress disorders result from major life stressors like divorce or a new job. The possibility of stressors should be elicited in the history.

Patients with chronic affective disorders have the same level of symptoms even in the follicular phase.

4. **A baby has just been delivered in the labour ward with ambiguous looking genitalia. Baby is otherwise normal. You are the registrar on duty.**

a. **What advice will you give the parents regarding the condition?**
(6 marks)

Handle the couple sympathetically and reassure them that the baby is otherwise healthy but the sex organs have not yet developed completely. The external genital organs are modified in such a way that we are unable to assign a specific gender to this baby as yet. _3 marks_

This could have happened due to either a chromosomal disorder or more commonly because of endocrine abnormalities. At times these things can be difficult to diagnose and in the absence of any other structural malformation in the baby the ultrasound is unable to detect the situation. _2 marks_

We need to investigate this baby urgently as certain conditions unless promptly treated, may turn life-threatening. _1 mark_

b. **Enumerate the differential diagnosis.** **(4 marks)**

The prime diagnosis that needs to be ruled out is congenital-adrenal hyperplasia (CAH) because this is the only condition that is life threatening. _2 marks_

Differential diagnosis is broadly divided into four main categories:

Female pseudohermaphroditism, male pseudohermaphroditism, true hermaphroditism and gonadal dysgenesis. _2 marks_

c. **How will you investigate and manage the baby?** **(10 marks)**

Examine the baby to find out if gonads are palpable (most important-if no gonads are palpable, baby is likely to be a girl), phallus length and diameter, position of urinary meatus, and the degree of labioscrotal fusion. Find out if there is a vagina, vaginal pouch or urogenital sinus. _2 marks_

Pelvic ultrasound or MRI to locate the internal gonads. _1 mark_

Blood for karyotyping, serum electrolytes, androgens, 17-OHP, 11-deoxy-corticosterone and 11-deoxycortisol. _2 marks_

Laparoscopy, gonadal biopsy and/or gonadectomy may be required later in selected cases. _1 mark_

Management should take into account the diagnosis and parental wishes. It is better to delay sex assignment (can be done up to 18 months) rather than reversing it at a later date. _1 mark_

Multidisciplinary team should be involved in the neonates care.   1 mark

Prompt correction of electrolyte imbalance and cortisol for adrenocorticotropic hormone suppression are areas of immediate concern.   2 marks

IMPORTANT NOTE

The first diagnosis to be confirmed or refuted for such an infant is CAH. It is the commonest cause of a masculinised female and is due to deficiency of 21-hydroxylase enzyme which converts 17α-hydroxyprogesterone to deoxycortisol and progesterone to deoxycorticosterones.

The androgens which need to be measured in blood are androstenedione, testosterone, DHEA, and DHEAS.

The lab findings may be:
1. ***Female pseudohermaphroditism** (genetic females with excess androgens) in the absence of maternal androgen excess- three forms of congenital virilizing adrenal hyperplasia:*
   a. *21-Hydroxylase deficiency: Elevated serum 17 OHP. This is the commonest form of congenital adrenal hyperplasia, the most frequent cause for sexual ambiguity and the most frequent endocrine cause of neonatal death.*
   b. *11β-hydroxylase deficiency: Elevated serum 11-deoxycorticosterone and 11-deoxycortisol.*
   c. *3β-hydroxysteroid dehydrogenase deficiency: elevated 17-hydroxy-pregnanolone and dehydroepiandrosterone.*
2. ***True hermaphrodite or gonadal dysgenesis**: Normal androgens, normal 17-OHP. Gonadal biopsy is required to confirm the diagnosis.*

Time allowed: 1.45 hours   *MM 80*

1. You are the registrar on duty and the midwife in room no 4 sounds the emergency alarm. You rush to the room and find the baby's head is lying at the perineum and the midwife is struggling to deliver the shoulders.

   (15, 5 marks)

   a. What would be your immediate actions?
   b. Enumerate the predictors for shoulder dystocia.

2. A 40-year-old woman presents for her first antenatal visit at your office. She has had her embryos transferred three weeks back and has just confirmed her pregnancy. (14, 6 marks)

   a. Describe your plan of care for her pregnancy.
   b. She has heard about cord blood banking and wishes to discuss the same with you. She is not aware of any genetic disorders in the family. Provide guidelines of your counselling session with her.

3. A 53-year-old postmenopausal school teacher has been suffering from urinary incontinence for the last 5 years. (10, 10 marks)

   a. Discuss the relevant history and investigations that you would like to perform in order to arrive at a diagnosis.
   b. What are the treatment options?

4. A parous 25-year-old woman complains of break through bleeding whilst taking the combined pill for oral contraception. (8, 12 marks)

   a. What relevant history would you enquire about?
   b. How will you manage her?

1. **You are the registrar on duty and the midwife in room no 4 sounds the emergency alarm. You rush to the room and find the baby's head is lying at the perineum and the midwife is struggling to deliver the shoulders.**

a. **What would be your immediate actions?** **(15 marks)**

Help: Call the senior obstetrician, SHO, midwife coordinator, neonatal team and anaesthetist for help. Ask a junior midwife to note time of manoeuvres.   2 marks

Episiotomy: Perform or extend episiotomy to create space for performing manoeuvres. Move buttocks to the edge of table. Put your hand in the sacral hollow to find out the position of posterior shoulder.   2 marks

Legs: With the help of two assistants, perform exaggerated flexion of maternal hips (McRobert's manoeuvre) with slight adduction. This increases the anteroposterior diameter of maternal pelvis and may release the anterior shoulder without needing to do anything further.   2 marks

Pressure: Synchronise the maternal pushing with constant suprapubic pressure and gentle downward traction on the foetal head to force the anterior shoulder under the pubic symphysis.   2 marks

Enter: Place your finger behind the anterior shoulder and try to rotate them into oblique diameter. Sweep the posterior arm across the foetal chest. Attempt the Wood's corkscrew manoeuvres next by putting two fingers behind the posterior shoulder in an attempt to rotate it through 180 degree. Since, the pelvis is longer posteriorly, when the lower posterior shoulder reaches anteriorly, it becomes deliverable.   2 marks

Remove: Remove the posterior arm by grasping the forearm and sweep it across the chest.   1 mark

Roll: If there is no other option, manoeuvres can be repeated with the mother on all fours.   1 mark

If the baby is still alive, cleidotomy or symphysiotomy can be tried by experienced operators. Zavanelli's manoeuvre to replace the head back into maternal abdomen and then delivering the baby by caesarean section has been successful in a few cases.   2 marks

If the foetus dies during the manoeuvres, destructive procedures may be undertaken by an experienced operator.   1 mark

b. **Enumerate the predictors for shoulder dystocia.** **(5 marks)**

It is difficult to predict shoulder dystocia. Majority occurs in infants less than 4.5 kg.   2 marks

Maternal diabetes, foetal macrosomia, previous history of shoulder dystocia (Recurrence risk 10%), prolonged labour, and delay in second stage are strong risk factors.   3 marks

IMPORTANT INFORMATION

All the manoeuvres for correcting shoulder dystocia aim to increase the pelvic diameters and some reduce the biacromial diameter. Each manoeuvre should be undertaken for 30 to 60 seconds before moving on.

The Helperr mnemonic (look at the first alphabet of each paragraph) is often used as a memory aid in shoulder dystocia management.

After the delivery of head, pH of the umbilical cord drops by 0.04/min. Interval between head and trunk delivery should be within 5 min.

2. A 40-year-old woman presents for her first antenatal visit at your office. She has had her embryos transfered three weeks back and has just confirmed her pregnancy.

a. Describe your plan of care for her pregnancy. **(14 marks)**

Confirm the number of foetuses – single or multiple; with their cardiac activity and chorionicity by transvaginal scan between 5 to 6 weeks. Rule out the presence of any heterotrophic pregnancy. 2 marks

Luteal support should be continued till at least 9 weeks of pregnancy or longer depending on the local protocols. 2 marks

Adequate folic acid supplementation and baseline pregnancy investigation should already have been advised. 1 mark

Offer screening for Down's syndrome with an early anomaly scan to check for Nuchal translucency and Nasal bone between 11 to 13 weeks. If screen positive offer amn iocentesis/CVS. 3 marks
Offer anomaly scan between 18 to 20 weeks and a foetal echocardiography between 22 to 24 weeks. 2 marks

Monitor maternal blood pressure, blood sugar and foetal health by regular antenatal visits, and serial biometric growth scans for the foetus. If foetal growth is restricted serial Doppler waveform analysis should be done to ascertain the right time for delivery. 2 marks

If required, prophylactic antenatal steroids should be administered once before 34 weeks. 1 mark

Deliver in specialist unit with Neonatal ICU facilities and monitor CTG during labour. 1 mark

b. She has heard about cord blood banking and wishes to discuss the same with you. She is not aware of any genetic disorders in the family. Provide guidelines of your counselling session with her. **(6 marks)**

Cord blood is the baby's blood that remains in the placenta and umbilical cord after birth. This blood contains stem cells which can be used for future transplantation in children and young adults if required. This is known as cord blood or stem cell transplant. 1 mark

A cord blood transplant can treat a few blood, immune and metabolic diseases, most common being childhood leukemia's. 1 mark

Cord blood is not usually collected as a routine but it can be collected safely from the umbilical cord after delivery and stored in a cord blood bank for a possible future use. 1 mark

There are two types of cord blood banks in the UK: Public and commercial banks. Private Banks store cord blood for a possible future use by an individual's own family by charging a fee. Prior consent is required before the collection can be organised. 1 mark

The RCOG supports only public cord banking and donation to the NHS cord blood bank but remains unconvinced about the benefit of storing cord blood with a private bank for families who have no known medical reasons to do so. 1 mark

Provide her with information leaflet on Cord Blood Banking. 1 mark

3. A 53-year-old postmenopausal school teacher has been suffering from urinary incontinence for the last 5 years.

a. Discuss the relevant history and investigations that you would like to perform in order to arrive at a diagnosis. **(10 marks)**

A complete gynaecological, obstetric, medical, and surgical history should be elicited, including a history of chronic cough, smoking, constipation or uterocervical descent. These, if present, will need simultaneous correction. 1 mark

Review any past history of medical therapy for incontinence. Undertake a general, systemic and gynaecological examination to demonstrate stress urinary incontinence if present. 1 mark

A Q tip placed at the bladder neck, and watching its movements during coughing will indicate hyper mobility of the bladder neck. 1 mark

MSU examination should be undertaken to check the specific gravity of the urine which is low in diabetes insipidus or inappropriate ADH syndrome. Urine culture and sensitivity should be done to rule out urinary tract infection, which should be treated prior to any surgical intervention. 2 marks

Ultrasound of the lower abdomen will reveal any ureteric or vesical stones that can result in both urinary infection as well as urinary urgency. A post void volume check should be made on ultrasound scan which will exclude overflow incontinence. 2 marks

Urodynamic testing to exclude detrusor instability should be considered. 1 mark

Blood sugar should be done according to hospital protocols for detection of diabetes. 1 mark

Maintenance of a fluid intake/void diary will reveal the social incapacitation from incontinence and whether fluid restriction would help. 1 mark

b. What are the treatment options? **(10 marks)**

Treatment options depend on the type of incontinence. 1 mark

Most patients have either a mixed picture or genuine stress incontinence. These patients need to supplement bladder drill, Kegel's exercises, use of weighted vaginal cones, and vaginal oestrogen administration for urogenital atrophy prior to surgical correction. 2 marks

Medical management is the first line treatment in cases of detrusor instability. It consists of administration of parasympatholytics like oxybutanin, duloxetine and tolterodine. 1 mark

Options for surgical management consist of both abdominal and vaginal procedures. Burch colposuspension has been the procedure of choice in genuine stress incontinence. It gives an immediate cure rate of 90 per cent with a five-year cure rate of around 70 per cent. 2 marks

Recently transvaginal tape (TVT) and trans-obturator tape (TOT) which employ nonabsorbable proline mesh for lifting the urethrovesical junction have become popular. They have the advantage of being less invasive, require shorter anaesthesia and can be performed as day cases. In patients that are poor surgical candidates, i.e. diabetics and obese women, these procedures can be performed under local anaesthesia. In comparative studies they give an 80 to 85 per cent cure rate but long-term cure rate studies are still awaited. 1 mark

Repair of cystocoel and buttressing of bladder neck is not the procedure of choice when genuine stress incontinence is present as both the primary cure rate and the long-term cure rates are inferior to Burch colposuspension. 1 mark

Other less frequently performed surgical procedures are Pereyra's needle suspension, Marshall Marketi Krantz (which can cause osteitis pubis) and other sling procedures. 1 mark

Collagen injections around the urethral meatus can be done if there is a short and patulous urethral opening. Insertion of an artificial sphincter can be done by urogynaecologists in cases of failure of primary Burch colposuspension. 1 mark

4. A parous 25-year-old woman complains of break through bleeding whilst taking the combined pill for oral contraception.

a. What relevant history would you enquire about? (8 marks)

The management of patients with abnormal bleeding involves in determining when the bleeding occurs with respect to the oestrogen and progestogen phases of cycle. Enquire about the duration of flow and the amount of blood loss. 1 mark

Is there a possibility of pregnancy related complications? Could the bleeding be due to local causes like a cervical erosion, polyp or retained foreign body? 2 marks

Enquire about the type and dose of pill that she is taking as the 20 µg pill is commonly associated with break through bleeding. Is there anything to suggest poor compliance? It should be stressed that she needs to take them at a specific time of the day, every day to minimise hormonal fluctuations which can cause break through bleeding. 2 marks

Is she taking any other drug therapy? Intake of exogenous hormones, antibiotics, antitubercular treatment (rifampicin), warfarin, and antiepileptics can cause hepatic enzyme induction and early clearance of oestrogens. Diarrhoea, vomiting, inflammatory bowel disorders, malabsorption syndromes, postsurgical stress can reduce absorption of hormones. 2 marks

Dietary history and family history of endometrial cancers, and coagulation defects should be elicited. 1 mark

b. How will you manage her? (12 marks)

Patient should be counselled regarding the problem and management should be directed towards the cause. 2 marks

A pregnancy test should be offered if there is any suspicion on account of missed pills or decreased drug availability. 1 mark

A speculum and digital vaginal examination should be done to look for cervicitis, polyps, enlarged uterus suggestive of fibroids and any adnexal fullness. 1 mark

Trans-vaginal ultrasound scanning should detect endometrial polyps, fibroids and hyperplasia. 1 mark

Vaginal swabs should be taken in suspected cases of infection. 1 mark

A pipelle or vabra aspiration should be offered for suspicious endometrium. Cervical cytology/PAP smear should be taken if due. 2 marks

If no significant pathology is identified and compliance is assured the first step in management would be to increase the daily dose of oestrogen such that the endometrium is stabilised followed by administration of progestogen to allow a controlled withdrawal bleed. In the next cycle consider using combined pills with higher oestrogen content if patient earlier was on an ultra-low dose preparation.

3 marks

If patient wishes to change her choice of contraception(consider mirena), appropriate counselling in this regard about available options and the advantages and disadvantages of usage should be done.

1 mark

Time allowed: 1.45 hours   *MM 80*

1. A pregnant woman presents at the labour ward at 3 am with fresh bleeding per vaginum for the last 30 min. This is her easarean second pregnancy having delivered the first one four years back with a C-section for foetal distress. She is 24/40 and she has slight tachycardia.   (12, 8 marks)
   a. She gives history of similar episode last month which was managed conservatively. Her scan then showed the presence of a low lying anterior placenta praevia covering the internal os. Enumerate your actions in the next 30 min.
   b. Three days later she has another bout of heavy bleeding in the hospital and you decide to do an emergency section for her. What precautions should be taken to minimise morbidity?

2. a. Describe the indications for use of Anti-D in a woman. (16, 4 marks)
   b. Discuss the possible routes of administration of Anti-D.

3. A couple has been living together for 2 years and has been unable to have a baby even after having regular unprotected intercourse. They come to you for advice.   (11, 9 marks)
   a. Discuss the relevant history, examination and investigations that you will advice.
   b. Discuss the general advice that you will impart at this stage.

4. A 40-year-old woman having heavy periods for the last 10 years has been found to have a single intramural myoma of 43 mm × 37 mm, on sonography. She comes to you for advice.   (20 marks)
   What are the management options available to her?

1. **A pregnant woman presents at labour ward at 3 am with fresh bleeding per vaginum for the last 30 min. This is her second pregnancy having delivered the first one four years back with a C-section for foetal distress. She is 24/40 and she has slight tachycardia.**

a. **She gives history of similar episode last month which was managed conservatively. Her scan then showed the presence of a low lying anterior placenta praevia covering the internal os. Enumerate your actions in the next 30 min.** **(15 marks)**

Admit her in the hospital with access to the HDU. 1 mark

Inform the obstetric consultant and haematologist. 1 mark

Assess the estimated blood loss by history, visual inspection and status of pulse, blood pressure and pallor. Assign a dedicated midwife to record vital parameters, hourly urine output, fluids and drugs used. 2 marks

Secure intravenous access with two large bore 14 or 16 G cannulae. Start crystalloids. Withdraw 20 ml blood for urgent haematological investigations—full blood count, group and cross match, platelet and fibrinogen levels. 3 marks

Record pulse oxymetry and give oxygen by mask at 4 to 6 litres. 1 mark

Insert urinary catheter. 1 mark

Organise an urgent ultrasound scan for foetal cardiac activity and placentation. Look meticulously for evidence of morbidly adherent placenta with the aid of Doppler. 4 marks

If she is Rh negative, give her a normal dose of Anti D and order Kleihauer count. 1 mark

Administer first dose of antenatal steroids. 1 mark

b. **Three days later she has another bout of heavy bleeding in the hospital and you decide to do an emergency section for her. What precautions should be taken to minimise morbidity?** **(10 marks)**

Inform senior obstetric consultant, senior anaesthetist, neonatologist, theatre staff and NICU for readiness. 1 mark

General anaesthesia is preferable. 1 mark

Most senior member of the obstetric team to do the surgery as there possibility of excessive blood loss senior anaesthetist consultant should be present. 1 mark

Recheck consent for blood transfusion and a possible hysterectomy. 1 mark

Lower segment approach may be difficult due to big vessels. She may require a vertical or classical uterine incision. Avoid cutting or shearing the placenta to avoid foetal blood loss. If the placenta is morbidly adherent, no attempt should be made to separate it. The cord should be tied close to the placenta, and methotrexate 1 mg/kg may be injected into the cord vessels. Alternatively, Hysterectomy with placenta in situ may be performed.   3 marks

Prophylactic use of prostaglandin is recommended to decrease the blood loss.

1 mark

Commence broad spectrum prophylactic antibiotics to minimise sepsis. 1 mark

Meticulous documentation of case notes is essential.   1 mark

2. a. Describe the indications for use of Anti-D in a woman. (16 marks)

Anti-D immunoglobulin (Ig) is given to prevent alloimmunisation resulting from foeto maternal haemorrhages (FMHs) occurring in an RhD negative woman carrying an RhD positive foetus. 2 marks

Antenatally, at least 250 IU of Anti-D Ig should be given before 20 weeks' gestation and 1500 IU thereafter. A test for the size of FMH is preferable when anti-D Ig is given after 20 weeks and additional doses given, if required. It is used: 8 marks

- Before 12 weeks, if there has been uterine instrumentation. (Omit if no surgical intervention).
- Ectopic pregnancy.
- Termination of pregnancy at any time (medical or surgical).
- Spontaneous complete or incomplete abortion after 12 weeks of pregnancy.
- Threatened miscarriage after 12 weeks. If bleeding continues intermittently, after 12 weeks, repeat anti-D at 6 weekly intervals.
- If uterine bleeding is very heavy and gestation is approaching 12 weeks, Anti-D may be considered. Confirm period of gestation by ultrasound.
- Any time in pregnancy after the following potentially sensitising events;
  - Invasive prenatal diagnosis (amniocentesis, chorionic villus sampling, foetal blood sampling).
  - Other intrauterine procedures (e.g. insertion of shunts, embryo reduction).
  - Ante partum haemorrhage.
  - External cephalic version of the foetus.
  - Closed abdominal injury.
  - Intrauterine death.
- Routine antenatal prophylaxis at 28 and 34 weeks with 1500 IU (300 microgram) decreases the incidence of alloimmunisation from 99.2 to 99.7 percent.

Postnatally: At least 1500 IU of anti-D Ig must be given to every non-sensitised RhD negative woman within 72 hours following the delivery of an RhD positive infant. This includes women with alloantibodies other than anti-D. 1500 IU of anti-D Ig is capable of suppressing immunisation by up to 15 ml of RhD positive red cells. Kleihauer Betke Test to detect FMH greater than 4 ml must also be undertaken, so that additional anti-D Ig can be given as appropriate. 3 marks

If a woman has received injection anti-D during pregnancy, she may have detectable anti-D in her blood at delivery, anti-D Ig should be given to such women unless it has been clearly confirmed that she is already sensitised. 1 mark

Therapeutic use: If an RhD negative woman requires platelet transfusion, RhD negative platelets should be transfused. If it is necessary to transfuse RhD positive platelets anti-D prophylaxis with 250 IU (50 micrograms) should be given after every 3 adult doses of platelets as there may be some contamination from red cells (< 0.1 ml RBC per vac). 2 marks

b. Discuss the possible routes of administration of Anti-D. (4 marks)

It is routinely administered as *Intramuscular* injections, best given into the deltoid muscle, (injections into the gluteal region often only reach the subcutaneous tissues and absorption may be delayed). 1 mark

Patients having marked thrombocytopaenia should be given the anti-D Ig *subcutaneously* to avoid the possibility of a haematoma following intramuscular injection. 1 mark

Intravenous anti-D Ig is the preparation of choice when large volumes of Rh-positive blood has been transfused. Intramuscular anti-D Ig must not be given intravenously. 1 mark

Exchange transfusion may be considered after adequate patient counselling when more than 2 units of RhD positive blood have been transfused. 1 mark

IMPORTANT INFORMATION

Anti-D use can be divided into prophylactic and therapeutic use. Further subdivision into usual and unusual dosage and route of administration can be planned. Use during Antenatal or postnatal period should be discussed. 99.2 to 99.3 percent women in UK have fetomaternal haemorrhage (FMH) <4 ml at delivery. Up to 50% of larger FMHs occur after normal deliveries without any overt sensitising event. Kleihauer acid elution test to detect fetal hemoglobin (Hb F), flow cytometry to detect RhD positive red cells or rosetting technique can be employed to detect FMH. Anticoagulated blood collected within 2 hours of the event should be used.

Anti-D is a blood product and women, especially Jehovah's Witness must make an informed decision prior to use.

Anti-D Ig should be given intramuscularly as soon as possible and within 72 hours after the sensitising event. If it is not given before 72 hours, a dose given within 9 to 10 days may provide some protection. Beyond 28 days, it loses its protection Women who are already sensitised or have a weak expression of RhD (Du) should not be given anti-D Ig.

3. **A couple has been living together for 2 years and has been unable to have a baby even after having regular unprotected intercourse. They come to you for advice.**

a. **Discuss the relevant history, examination and investigations that you will advise.** **(11 marks)**

A need and risk assessment should be done by eliciting a history covering life style, frequency of intercourse, sexual, obstetrical and contraceptives in a sensitive manner. 2 marks

General physical examination, including height, weight, and BMI should be measured. Presence of galactorrhoea should be looked for. 1 mark

Pelvic examination for presence of vaginal discharge, uterine fibroids and adnexal masses should be done. 1 mark

In the absence of any obvious problem, provide reassurance as spontaneous conception rates are 90 to 95 per cent within 3 years of unprotected intercourse (for women <35 years) and initiate basic investigations. The couple's assessment of perceived problem should be taken into account and they should be allowed to make an informed decision regarding their management. 2 marks

Initial investigations like semen analysis for the male partner, assessment of ovulation and tubal patency for the female partner should be advised. Screening for cervical chlamydial infection should be offered as treatment of the same can decrease the incidence of pelvic infection and related infertility. 2 marks

Tests for ovulation assessment include day 21 or mid luteal serum progesterone and follicular study by transvaginal sonography. If anovulatory then serum prolactin, thyroid function and pituitary gonadotropins should be checked. 2 marks

In the absence of known pelvic pathology hyterosalpingogram (HSG) remains the investigation of choice for judging the tubal patency if pelvic ultrasound and ovulation tests are normal. 1 mark

b. **Discuss the general advice that you will impart at this stage.** **(9 marks)**

Changes in lifestyle should be advised which include; regular sexual intercourse every 2 to 3 days, limiting alcohol intake to ≤ 1 to 2 unit's alcohol/week for women; ≤ 3-4/ week for men, and maintaining the BMI of both partners close to 19 to 25. Men should avoid tight fitting under clothing for prolonged period of time. 2 marks

They should be advised to avoid both active and passive smoking. Referral to a smoking cessation program may be offered. Use of recreational drugs and other medications should be enquired. Marijuana is a major cause of decreased sperm count. 2 marks

Appropriate Folic acid supplementation should be prescribed for at least 3 months. Rubella status should be checked and if susceptible rubella vaccination offered. Avoid pregnancy for at least one month after vaccination. If relevant cervical screening should be offered. 3 marks

Women with known predisposing factors for infertility should be referred to specialist centres and offered extended counselling. Information leaflets should be provided and if required help with contact numbers of support group agencies may be provided. 2 marks

IMPORTANT NOTE

All couples with inability to conceive after 2 years of regular unprotected intercourse should be offered investigations. They can be initiated even after one year if age of the female partner is ≥ 35 years or they have an identifiable cause. Cause of infertility is – unidentified in 30 per cent couples.

Ovulatory disorders in 27 per cent
Tubal damage in 14 per cent
Male factor in 19 per cent
Both male and female factors in 39 per cent

HSG is a reliable indicator of tubal patency but not of occlusion. Hence, it is used as a screening test in couples with no history of pelvic infection and if abnormal, confirmatory laparoscopy should follow. It is also less invasive and cost-effective than laparoscopy.

Chlamydial infection can cause both male and female infertility. PCR is currently the test of choice for diagnosis. Confirmed cases require treatment with Doxycycline, partner notification, contact tracing and referral to genitourinary clinics.

Effects of drugs/toxins on male infertility include:
- *Sulfa drugs – impaired spermatogenesis*
- *Narcotics – decreased libido*
- *Phenytoin – ejaculatory dysfunction*
- *Diethylstillbesterol – testicular atrophy*
- *Radiotherapy – germ cell depletion*

4. **A 40-year-old woman having heavy periods for the last 10 years has been found to have a single intramural myoma of 43 mm × 37 mm, on sonography. She comes to you for advice.**

   What are the management options available to her?   **(20 marks)**

Symptoms like pain, intermenstrual bleeding and pressure symptoms which may be associated with fibroids along with the fertility aspirations of the woman should be known prior to giving her the options.   2 marks

Other causes of heavy bleeding especially those related to intrauterine devices and infection should be ruled out after abdominal, speculum and bimanual examinations.   2 marks

Complete blood count including platelet count, thyroid function tests and coagulation tests should be performed if there is any positive history.   2 marks

If her heavy cycles are not influencing her general health and lifestyle, and if asymptomatic otherwise, she should be kept under surveillance provided FBC is normal.   2 marks

Appropriate Medical management with Mefanemic acid and Tranexamic acid should be offered for menorrhagia along with haematinics, if required. 2 marks

If symptomatic menorrhagia or reproductive failure is a problem, Myomectomy may be offered. In cases of intramural myomas with a submucous component, hysteroscopic myomectomy is superior, if expertise exists. Haemorrhage, infection, chance of scar dehiscence during subsequent pregnancy, and recurrence are common complications. It should be offered if she desires to preserve her uterus for future reproduction.   2 marks

Levonorgestral—releasing intrauterine system (Mirena) is effective in decreasing fibroid related menorrhagia provided the uterine cavity is not distorted. It may also cause fibroid shrinkage.   2 marks

GnRH analogues have a high incidence of adverse effects and should not be used for more than 6 months. They should be used selectively to reduce fibroid volume and control excessive bleeding preoperatively. Add – back treatment should be considered.   2 marks

Uterine artery embolisation, laparoscopic myolysis, high intensity focused ultrasound (HIFU), MRI-guided laser ablation and laser photocoagulation are newer techniques for treatment of symptomatic fibroids in women not desiring further childbirth. Some of these techniques are still undergoing clinical trials.   2 marks

Hysterectomy provides definitive cure to symptomatic women who have completed their family. It is desirable to perform through the vaginal route with laparoscopic assistance.   2 marks

IMPORTANT NOTE

Fibroids are present in 25 per cent of women during reproductive age group.

Time allowed: 1.45 hours   *MM 80*

1. A primigravid woman has been referred to your clinic with breech presentation at 37 weeks.   (6, 7, 7 marks)
    a. How would you counsel her about the baby's presentation?
    b. What are the management options available to her for delivery?
    c. She wishes to try External Cephalic Version. What information would you provide her with?

2. An ultrasound scan performed following raised alpha-fetoprotein (AFP) at 16 weeks gestation reveals an anterior abdominal defect in the foetus.   (6, 14 marks)
    a. She wishes to know about the conditions that may be associated with raised AFP.
    b. How will you counsel the parents and manage the rest of the pregnancy?

3. A 25-year-old woman of Asian origin requests an abortion citing personal reasons. She is 8 weeks pregnant.   (15, 5 marks)
    a. Discuss her management.
    b. Describe the relevant post procedure issues.

4. A 24-year-old woman presents at A and E to seek advice. She has missed her oral contraceptive pills and is now worried.   (20 marks)
    What information would you ask for and give?

1. A primigravid woman has been referred to your clinic with breech presentation at 37 weeks.

a. How would you counsel her about the baby's presentation? **(6 marks)**

Breech means that the baby is lying bottom first or feet first in the womb (uterus) instead of in the usual head first position. In early pregnancy, breech is very common. As pregnancy continues, a baby usually turns by itself into the head first position but at present, your baby has not done so. Four per cent of all singleton pregnancies are breech presentations. **1 mark**

Such babies are sometimes at a higher risk of congenital malformations and cerebral palsy. These risks are higher in preterm babies but there is no evidence from ultrasound scans that your baby may be having any such problems. **2 marks**

Since the baby's head has not got used to the birth passage, there might be problems to you and baby during delivery and we may have to adopt different ways to deliver this baby safely. **1 mark**

Inform her about the various options for delivery and allow the couple to make an informed decision. **1 mark**

Appropriate documentation of the counselling and women's decision should be made in her case records. Provide her with an information leaflet. **1 mark**

b. What are the management options available to her for delivery?
(7 marks)

Recent ultrasound (after 36 weeks) should be rechecked to confirm presentation, rule out placenta praevia and foetal malformations. Adequacy of liquor, attitude of limbs (flexed, extended or footling) and head should be checked before giving her options. **1 mark**

She should be offered **External Cephalic Version (ECV)** by appropriately trained professionals at 38 weeks. **1 mark**

Postural management to promote cephalic version include knee chest position and elevation of pelvis using a cushion. It is popular but not very effective. RCOG does not recommend it. **1 mark**

Elective caesarean section at 39 weeks is now considered the safest mode of delivery for a singleton, uncomplicated breech baby (Term breech trial). The chances of neonatal respiratory morbidity and mortality are decreased and there is a small chance of spontaneous correction of lie till that time. She still has around 70 per cent chance of normal vaginal delivery in her next pregnancy. **2 marks**

The inherent risks of a surgical procedure, especially thromboembolism, bleeding and infection should be explained. If spontaneous labor starts before the scheduled surgery, emergency CS may be required; this may carry a higher morbidity.

1 mark

Trial of vaginal delivery may be offered in the absence of any medical or obstetric complications. It carries higher risks of foetal morbidity and mortality and 20 per cent women may still require emergency CS due to various reasons. If she still chooses to deliver vaginally or presents in advance labour, appropriately trained personnel should be present to conduct delivery.

1 mark

c. **She wishes to try External Cephalic Version. What information would you provide her with?** **(7 marks)**

Vaginal breech birth is more complicated than normal birth. We may try and turn the baby to a head first position by applying gentle pressure on your abdomen so the baby somersaults to lay head first. This technique is called External Cephalic version or ECV. This increases the likelihood of having a vaginal birth.

1 mark

It would be performed on the labour ward, near to the facilities for emergency delivery. ECV carries a success rate of 40 to 60 per cent and halves the rates of caesarean sections done for breech presentation. If you find it uncomfortable, you can ask for pain relief or to stop the procedure.

2 marks

Less than 1 per cent women will require emergency caesarean section for procedure related foetal distress, placental abruption and vaginal bleeding. Appropriate doses of injection Anti-D (after Kleihauer count) would be administered if required.

1 mark

It would be done under ultrasound guidance. Cardiotocography (CTG) before and after ECV, reconfirms foetal well being. Relaxing the muscles of the womb (Tocolysis) is likely to improve chances of success.

1 mark

If the baby does not want to turn, it is possible to have a second attempt on another day. If the baby does not turn after a second attempt, we may have to proceed with an alternative method of delivery.

1 mark

She should telephone the hospital if she has bleeding, abdominal pain, contractions or reduced movements after ECV.

1 mark

IMPORTANT INFORMATION

The commonest reason of a breech presentation is prematurity.

Moxibustion is not a standard practice but is known to be safe and may promote spontaneous version.

It refers to burning of special herbs to stimulate the acupuncture points beside the outer corner of fifth toenail.

Contraindications to ECV include women in active labour, twins, extended foetal head, uterine scar or abnormality, foetal compromise, ruptured membranes, placenta praevia, vaginal bleeding and medical conditions.

2. **An ultrasound scan performed following raised alpha-foetoprotein (AFP) at 16 weeks gestation reveals an anterior abdominal defect in the foetus.**

a. **She wishes to know about the conditions that may be associated with raised AFP.** **(6 marks)**

The commonest conditions associated with a raised AFP are neural tube defects like open spina bifida, encephalocoel and anencephaly. 2 marks

Foetal conditions like abdominal wall defects, renal disorders, i.e. congenital nephrosis, uropathies, bowel obstruction, sacrococcygeal teratoma and skin disorders may be associated with it. 2 marks

Pregnancy related complications like growth restriction, foetomaternal haemorrhage; oligohydramnios, preterm membrane rupture and placental tumours may be co-existent. 1 mark

Gestation more advanced than suspected, extremes of maternal weight and multiple pregnancies will show erroneously high values. 1 mark

b. **How will you counsel the parents and manage the rest of the pregnancy?** **(14 marks)**

Parents should be dealt sympathetically and the differential diagnosis of such defects should be informed, i.e. gastroschisis, omphalocoele and hernia. 1 mark

Omphalocoele (exomphalos) is an abdominal wall hernia due to arrest of ventral medial migration of dermatomyotomes. Sixty to eighty per cent foetuses are associated with structural (esp. cardiac) or chromosomal anomalies. One in six babies will have abnormal karyotype but for normal karyotypic foetuses, survivability is around 75 per cent. 2 marks

Further investigations, such as detailed ultrasound and foetal echo-cardiography should be arranged. Karyotyping should be offered. 2 marks

Termination of pregnancy is an appropriate option before viability. 1 mark

Gastroschisis is a Para–umbilical defect of the anterior abdominal wall, usually considered a developmental accident. Less than 10 per cent foetuses have associated anomalies, and only 1 per cent have abnormal karyotype. The chances of a good outcome are very high with over 80 per cent survival. 2 marks

Serial ultrasound scans after 24 weeks to assess foetal growth, amniotic fluid volume and bowel appearance should be arranged. 1 mark

Parents should be offered extended counselling sessions with a multi-disciplinary team comprising of an obstetrician with expertise in foetal medicine, a neonatal poediatrician, poediatric surgeon, clinical geneticist and anaesthetist if they decide to continue pregnancy. They will all decide the outline of management once the baby is born.   1 mark

Information leaflets and illustrations showing pre- and post-surgery defects should be used at these sessions. Parents should be informed that baby may require prolonged hospital stay (up to 3 months) after birth and will require surgery to close the defect.   2 marks

Delivery should take place in a tertiary foetomaternal unit with neonatal surgical facilities. Inducing preterm labour is not indicated and vaginal delivery is usually appropriate in the absence of medical or obstetric complications.   1 mark

Parents should be offered a lot of psychological support and informed that the risk of recurrence for the next pregnancy is usually low, i.e. less than 1 per cent.
                                                                                        1 mark

IMPORTANT INFORMATION

Alpha foetoprotein is a glycoprotein similar to albumin. It is synthesised initially in foetal yolk sac and then foetal liver.

Foetal serum alpha foetoprotein concentration peaks at 13 weeks and it enters the amniotic fluid via foetal urination. After that the foetal values decline. From the amniotic fluid, it diffuses across the placenta and amnion.

The maternal serum values (MSAFP) continues to rise till 30 to 32 weeks before declining.

Insulin dependent diabetic mothers have lower MSAFP but four times the incidence of NTD than non-diabetic mothers.

3. **A 25-year-old woman of Asian origin requests an abortion citing personal reasons. She is 8 weeks pregnant.**

a. **Discuss her management.** **(15 marks)**

Both medical and surgical methods are safe, effective and acceptable at this gestational age. 1 mark

If the gestational age or location is doubtful, a scan should be offered to determine the same. She should be informed that the earlier in pregnancy an abortion is performed, the lesser are the complication rates. 2 marks

Testing for haemoglobin concentration, ABO and rhesus blood groups, red cell antibodies, and HIV should be performed. Testing for haemoglobinopathies, vaginal swabs for Chlamydia and hepatitis B, and C should be offered in the presence of high-risk factors. 3 marks

Adequate counselling should be offered and information leaflets provided so that she can make an informed decision regarding the options available. A language interpreter and a chaperone should preferably be present. 3 marks

Medical abortion using mifepristone plus prostaglandin is appropriate till 9 weeks gestational age (63 days). Mifepristone 200 mg orally followed 1 to 3 days later by gemeprost 0.5 mg or misoprostol 400 mg vaginally is the recommended regimen. The success rate is close to 95 per cent and 1 per cent women continued pregnancy requiring a second trial with medical abortion or proceeding to surgical termination. 2 marks

Suction termination is usually done under general anaesthesia (GA) but local anaesthesia (Para-cervical block) is safer than GA and may be offered. 1 marks

Cervical preparation with misoprostol (400 micrograms administered vaginally 3 hours before surgery) reduces the complication rate. Risk of uterine perforation (0.4%), hemorrhage (0.1%), cervical trauma, failed abortion necessitating further procedure should be informed. A small risk of hysterectomy must also be mentioned on the consent form. 2 marks

Electric or manual aspiration with special devices is effective, safe and has shorter operating time. 1 mark

b. **Describe the relevant post procedure issues.** **(5 marks)**

Anti D immunoglobulin 250 IU should be given to all RhD negative women within 72 hours following abortion, whether by surgical or medical means. 1 mark

Inform her in writing that she should contact the emergency services in case of excessive pain, bleeding or fever. Facilities for emergency admission should be available at all times. 1 mark

A discharge card containing details of the procedure performed should be provided before discharge. 1 mark

Advice for future contraception should be given. An intrauterine contraceptive can be inserted prior to discharge. 1 mark

A follow-up visit should be scheduled after 2 weeks. Another appointment may be arranged, if the woman wants further counselling. 1 mark

IMPORTANT NOTE

In UK, abortion is legal up to 24 weeks. For first 7 weeks, medical abortion is the first line method.

Terminations done after 12 weeks require the signature of two registered practitioners on the abortion form, but are seldom done for only social reasons. TOP for lethal abnormality can be done at any time before 24 weeks.

Medical pills should be avoided in women with suspected ectopic pregnancy, undiagnosed adnexal masses, intrauterine device in place, long-term systemic corticosteroid therapy, chronic adrenal failure, severe anaemia and known allergy. Misoprostol should be avoided in women with uncontrolled epilepsy and allergy to prostaglandin.

The risk of haemorrhage during a surgical evacuation is low; 1 in 1000.

Risk of uterine perforation is moderate; 1 to 4 in 1000.

Risk of cervical trauma and injury to cervical os is 1 in 100.

4. **A 24-year-old woman presents at A and E to seek advice. She has missed her oral contraceptive pills and is now worried.**

What information would you ask for and give? **(20 marks)**

1. When did she miss the pills? 1 mark

If the missed pill was scheduled at 12 hour or less, advise her to take the missed pill now and further pills as usual. 1 mark

If she has skipped it for more than 12 hour, she should take the most recent pill now and discard any earlier missed pills. She should use extra precaution (barriers) or abstain from intercourse for the next seven days. 2 marks

2. When did she begin the pack and how many tablets are left in the pack? 1 mark

If less than seven pills are remaining in the pack, she should finish that pack and start the next packet without the usual seven day pill free interval. Emergency contraception is not required if there is no Pill free interval (PFI). 2 marks

If more than seven pills are there in the pack, she should finish this pack and continue as usual with the next pack. 2 marks

3. How many tablets has she missed? 1 mark

If she has missed one or two 30 to 35 µg or one 20 µg ethinylestradiol (EE) pills, at any time, she should take the most recent missed pill as soon as possible and then continue taking the remaining pills daily, one each day, at her usual time. Additional or emergency contraception is not required. 3 marks

If 2 and more 20 µg or 3 and more 30 to 35 µg EE pills have been missed at any time during the cycle, she should take the most recent pill as soon as possible and then continue taking rest of the pills daily. Additional precautions like condoms or abstinence should be taken till she has taken pills for 7 days. 3 marks

If these pills are missed in week 1 (1-7 days of starting the pack), effectively extending the pill free interval and she had unprotected sex (in week 1 or in the PFI), emergency contraception should be considered. 2 marks

If she has missed more than seven active consecutive pills, then she must be viewed as having stopped taking the pill and the missed pills rules cannot be applied. 2 marks

IMPORTANT NOTE

COCs inhibit ovulation by reducing gonadotropins. They also make cervical mucus and endometrium hostile for implantation. Seven consecutive pills are regularly missed in the PFI without losing contraceptive protection. Follicular activity occurs

without ovulation in the PFI. Risk of failure is higher with combined oral contraceptives (COCs) containing low dose estrogens.

The chances of failure (pregnancy) depend on the **'Number'** of missed pills and also on **'When'** those pills are missed. The risk of pregnancy is greatest when pills are missed at the beginning or end of the pack containing active hormonal pills. Seven consecutive pills are required to inhibit ovulation and the rest for maintaining anovulation.

In UK, 21 day pill regimen (without the 7 inactive placebo pills) is commonly followed and advice is given accordingly.

Time allowed: 1.45 hours   *MM 80*

1. An epileptic woman controlled on carbamezapine and valproate wants
   to conceive and comes to you for advice.   (8, 12 marks)
   a. How will you counsel her?
   b. Briefly outline her antenatal and post-natal care.

2. A woman has just been admitted to the labour ward with confirmed
   spontaneous rupture of the membranes at 25 weeks gestation. Ultrasound
   reveals a singleton, healthy foetus in transverse lie at present.
   Describe your further management.   (20 marks)

3. A healthy 75-year-old woman has developed symptomatic vaginal vault
   prolapse many years after total abdominal hysterectomy for a benign
   pathology.   (12, 8 marks)
   a. What are her treatment options?
   b. She decides to undergo sacrocolpopexy with mesh repair. What are
      the specific complications of the procedure and how can they be
      minimised?

4. A 37-year-old woman presents at your OPD with slight vaginal bleeding.
   She has conceived with IVF and two embryos were transferred 6 weeks
   back. Transvaginal ultrasound shows an intrauterine pregnancy with a 7
   mm foetus but no foetal heart pulsations.
   How will you manage her?   (20 marks)

1. **An epileptic woman controlled on carbamezapine and valproate wants to conceive and comes to you for advice.**

a. **How will you counsel her?**   **(8 marks)**

Conception should be delayed till epilepsy is well controlled and medical optimisation has been achieved. If she has been seizure free for many years, reassure as majority (>50%) have a normal outcome. Twenty five per cent women may experience an increased frequency of seizures in pregnancy.   2 marks

There is no increased risk of miscarriage or obstetric complications due to epilepsy *per se* and there is no evidence of adverse effects of a single seizure on the foetus. Continuous seizures may cause hypoxia of the foetus.   1 mark

She should be advised to take 4 mg folic acid starting at least one month pre-conceptionaly till the end of pregnancy to counter the antifolate action of anti-convulsant drugs.   1 mark

Neuro physician involvement should be sought to review necessity of anticonvulsant drugs and if possible to put her on monotherapy at lowest possible doses.   1 mark

Risk of congenital malformations (GCA) should be discussed. Valproate (2%) and carbamezapine (1%) both can cause neural tube defects. Risk of GCA is higher (15%) with two drugs as compared to when she is controlled on single drug (6-7%). For valproate there is evidence of a dose-dependent teratogenic effect.   2 marks

Risk of epilepsy in offspring should be explained and genetic counselling offered.
                                                                     1 mark

b. **Briefly outline her antenatal and post-natal care.**   **(12 marks)**

During her **antenatal** period risk of seizures, its implications for license and social security and the importance of compliance with medication and folic acid should be stressed.   2 marks

If required, monitor free drug levels; advise good diet, sleep and avoidance of precipitating factors. Treat nausea and vomiting early.   1 mark

In second trimester, get a maternal serum Alfa-feto-protein level and detailed anomaly scan at 18 to 20 weeks. Consider amniocentesis.   1 mark

Offer multidisciplinary input with regular antenatal visits.   1 mark

In third trimester begin NST every week after 34 weeks and arrange regular growth scans if poorly controlled epileptic.   2 marks

Add oral vitamin K 10 mg/day in the last 4 weeks to decrease the risk of haemorrhagic disease of newborn. 1 mark

Post-natally neonate should also receive injection vitamin K. 1 mark

Encourage breastfeeding but monitor for signs of neonatal withdrawal or sedative effects. If present advise breastfeeding during the nadir drug concentration period, avoiding feeding during peak drug levels. 1 mark

If possible, reduce the dose of anticonvulsants gradually over 2 to 3 months. Avoid sleep deprivation and advice about avoidance of seizure related accidents.
1 mark

Contraception with higher doses of estrogens (50 to 100 μgm) in combined pills is desirable. Efficacy of progesterone pill may be affected by hepatic enzyme inducers like carbamezapine. Barriers, mirena (progesterone IUD) and progesterone injections are effective options. 1 mark

IMPORTANT NOTES

Valproate, clonazepam and newer drugs like vigabatrin, lamotrigine and gabapentin do not induce hepatic enzymes and all methods of contraception are suitable.

2 A woman has just been admitted to the labour ward with confirmed spontaneous rupture of the membranes at 25 weeks gestation. Ultrasound reveals a singleton, healthy foetus in transverse lie at present. Describe your further management. **(20 marks)**

Expectant management is the most favoured for premature rupture of membranes (PROM) between 24 to 31 weeks. 2 marks

A perspeculum examination to assess the cervix and to take culture swabs.

1 mark

Avoid digital vaginal examinations to assess cervical status unless labour is established in order to prevent the increased risk of ascending infection. 1 mark

Perform baseline tests for foetal and maternal well-being. 1 mark

Vigilance for chorioamnionitis should be maintained clinically (maternal fever, tachycardia, uterine pain/tenderness, purulent vaginal discharge) and by laboratory investigations (total and differential leukocyte count, C-reactive protein, amniotic fluid gram-stain, microscopy and culture). High vaginal swab should be taken at presentation and a wet preparation for Nugent scoring to look for bacterial vaginosis. 2 marks

Serial tests for foetal well-being; daily CTG, twice weekly biophysical profile, weekly liquor volume and Doppler studies, fortnightly growth scans should be undertaken.

2 marks

An early aggressive broad spectrum intravenous antibiotic therapy is essential. It causes a significant reduction in perinatal mortality and morbidity, together with a reduction in maternal infectious morbidity and an improvement in latency to delivery. 1 mark

A course of corticosteroids to induce foetal lung maturity is recommended in the absence of infection. 1 mark

Tocolytics such as nifedipine should be used until time is gained for corticosteroids to act or to facilitate fetomaternal transfer to tertiary center. 2 marks

Pregnancy should be continued till signs of chorioamnionitis or foetal distress develop. 1 mark

Home management is increasingly seen as a safe protocol to adopt, particularly if there is no evidence of infection and onset of labour after one week of PROM and ultrasound shows adequate amniotic fluid volume. Parents should be counselled regarding fetomaternal monitoring and the likely mode of delivery, if expectant management is not considered appropriate. 2 marks

Vaginal delivery is preferred except for breech presentation before 32 weeks. Caesarean section is reserved for usual obstetric indications. Outcome is improved if delivered in a center with good neonatal facilities. Paediatrician should be present at the time of delivery. 2 marks

After delivery neonate should be screened for evidence of sepsis. 1 mark

In the absence of a known aetiology the recurrence risk is as high as 20 to 30 per cent. 1 mark

IMPORTANT NOTE

The objective of management before 31 weeks of pregnancy is to prolong pregnancy if there are no signs of foetal or maternal infection as the risks due to prematurity far outweigh the risks of subclinical infection.

Between 31 to 36 weeks the management focus is balanced between preventing infectious morbidity and that due to pre-maturity.

Nearly half of the babies born before 26 weeks gestation will have some form of disability (cerebral palsy, mental retardation) and, in 50% of these the disability will be severe (EPICURE study).

3. **A healthy 75-year-old woman has developed symptomatic vaginal vault prolapse many years after total abdominal hysterectomy for a benign pathology.**

a. **What are her treatment options?** (12 marks)

Treatment options depend on her history, examination, discomfort and associated symptoms. Her present sexual history and desire for medical or surgical intervention should be known. 2 marks

Recurrent surgery is more complex, risky and prone to failure. She should be allowed to make an informed decision regarding her treatment. 1 mark

Conservative management includes use of shelf pessaries. HRT and physiotherapy are of little benefit. 1 mark

McCall's culdoplasty performed vaginally is an effective option. Uterosacral ligaments are identified and fixed to the pubocervical and rectovaginal fascia at the level of ischial spine. There is a one in 10 chance of ureteric damage and procedure is difficult with complete vault evertions. 2 marks

Sacrospinous fixation performed vaginally has high success rate, short hospital stay and less morbidity. It involves fixing the vagina with sacrospinous ligament but may cause pudendal nerve damage. 2 marks

Sacrocolpopexy requires an abdominal approach, longer operating time and hospital stay. There is risk of ureteric and bowel damage but is considered more effective. Laparoscopic approach should be offered if the expertise exists. 2 marks

Intravaginal slingplasty is a new day care procedure wherein a polypropylene tape is secured to the vagina and uterosacral ligaments. Long-term effectiveness studies are awaited. 1 mark

Colpocleisis is an option if she does not require a functional vagina. It may not be very suitable for healthy women. If genuine stress incontinence is identified, colposuspension may also be considered. 1 mark

b. **She decides to undergo sacrocolpopexy with mesh repair. What are the specific complications of the procedure and how can they be minimized? (8 marks)**

Intra-operative haemorrhage from presacral venous plexus or median sacral vessels can be prevented by using the sacral promontory instead of sacral hollow to attach the mesh. 3 marks

Ten per cent rate of mesh erosion can be minimised by the use of single flap mesh and attaching the mesh to pubocervical fascia anteriorly and rectovaginal fascia posteriorly instead of at the vaginal apex which may be devascularised.   3 marks

Constipation occurs due to rectal denervation and can be reduced by careful tissue handling.   1 mark

Stress urinary incontinence can be reduced with tension free application of mesh.
                                                                                                1 mark

4. **A 37-year-old woman presents at your OPD with slight vaginal bleeding. She has conceived with IVF and two embryos were transferred 6 weeks back. Transvaginal ultrasound shows an intrauterine pregnancy with a 7 mm foetus but no foetal heart pulsations.**
   How will you manage her?   **(20 marks)**

Foetal heart pulsations should be detectable in a foetus ≥ 6 mm or at 6 weeks. Since in an IVF pregnancy, the gestational age is certain, these findings suggest a failing pregnancy.   3 marks

While explaining the diagnosis to her, the term miscarriage should be used preferably instead of "abortion". The couple should be offered sympathetic counselling and provided with information leaflets. Her blood group and Rhesus factor should be checked.   3 marks

Unless the bleeding becomes heavy, pelvic examination and repeat ultrasound scanning within 1 to 2 days is not beneficial. Immediate hospital admission is not essential and she should be allowed to make an informed decision. The options include—expectant management, medical therapy, or surgical evacuation.
                                                                      4 marks

Expectant management includes repeating ultrasound scan after 1 week or anytime the bleeding becomes heavy. She may expel products of conception spontaneously. It may reassure the woman for diagnosis and avoid the need for admission and GA. Serial β HCG levels may be offered to check the rising titres. Absolute bed-rest, progesterone or HCG supplements are not effective.   4 marks

Medical management with mifepristone and prostaglandin is the preferred option when she is psychologically prepared.   2 marks

Surgical curettage may be required if expectant management fails or with heavy bleeding. Anti-D immunoglobulin should be administered if she is RhD negative, nonsensitised and undergoes evacuation.   2 marks

Follow-up extended counselling should be offered as a failed IVF pregnancy is a big psychological setback for the woman.   2 mark

Time allowed: 1.45 hours   *MM 80*

1. A primigravida at 13 weeks/gestation presents at A and E with history of severe vomiting for the past one week. On examination she has tachycardia and dehydration.   (4, 12, 4 marks)
   a. What is the likely diagnosis? Briefly outline other differential diagnosis.
   b. Describe your management of the case.
   c. What are the complications that may arise out of her condition?

2. A nulliparous woman at 30 weeks gestation presents at the labour ward with a BP of 180/110 and ++ protienuria. She has epigastric pain and right upper quadrant tenderness.   (8, 8, 4 marks)
   a. Describe your immediate management of the case.
   b. After six hours, her proteinuria becomes +++, BP is 150/100 mm Hg and liver enzymes are raised. How will you manage her now?
   c. You have informed the woman that an emergency section has to be performed to prevent deterioration in her condition. The couple wishes to know the implications for the baby. Since your paediatric colleague is not available at present; you have been asked to talk to the couple. What will you tell them?

3. A 32-year-old parous woman complains of postcoital bleeding. She is anxious as she has heard that it could be a sign of cancer.
                                                                  (4, 6, 10 marks)
   a. What are the possible causes of such bleeding in her?
   b. What relevant history would you enquire about?
   c. Describe her management including the investigations.

4. An 18-year-old woman complains of painful periods. She is not sexually active.
   Discuss her management.   (20 marks)

1. A primigravida at 13 weeks gestation presents at A and E with history of severe vomiting for the past one week. On examination she has tachycardia and dehydration.

a. What is the likely diagnosis? Briefly outline other differential diagnosis.

(4 marks)

Hyperemesis gravidarum is the likely diagnosis.   1 mark

History and clinical examination should be directed towards assessing her hydration status and ruling out other pathology like pyelonephritis, hepatitis, pancreatitis, diabetic ketoacidosis, thyrotoxicosis, gastroenteritis, molar pregnancy and drug-induced vomiting.   3 marks-any six

b. Describe your management of the case.   **(12 marks)**

She should be offered admission. Day care management is an accepted option for mild cases.   1 mark

Investigations include; full blood count for haematocrit and white cell count blood urea and electrolytes, serum calcium, liver function and thyroid function tests (look for hyperthyroidism) in severe cases.   1 mark

Urinalysis to exclude urinary tract infection, ketonuria.   1 mark

Ultrasonography to exclude molar and multiple pregnancies.   1 mark

On admission her weight, pulse and blood pressure should be recorded. Any emesis causing drugs should be suspended temporarily.   1 mark

Keep her nil by mouth or only ice till vomiting is controlled. Multidisciplinary team may need to be involved in her care. Intravenous rehydration should be by normal saline or Hartmann's solution with added potassium chloride in each bottle. Thiamine 100 mg should be added weekly. Fluid and electrolyte regimens should be altered every day according to need.   2 marks

Attending staff should provide lots of encouragement, reassurance and psychological support.   1 mark

Antiemetics; 5HT3 receptor antagonists (ondansetron) are effective in reducing nausea and vomiting. Pyridoxine is more effective in reducing severity of nausea. Ginger and P6 acupressure are of proven benefit.   1 mark

Antacids, H2 receptor antagonists (ranitidine) and proton pump inhibitors (Omeprazole) may be added to prevent acid peptic disease.   1 mark

Severe hyperemesis refractory to standard treatment may require total parentral nutrition, and corticosteroids. Upper GI endoscopy may be considered to rule out acid peptic disease, and oesophageal reflux. 1 mark

Termination of pregnancy may be offered in select cases. 1 mark

c. What are the complications that may arise out of her condition?
(4 marks)

Maternal complications that can complicate hyperemesis are oesophageal tears, hematemesis and Mallory-Weiss syndrome, Wernicke's encephalopathy, Korsakoff's psychosis, seizure and paralysis secondary to hyponatremia and hepatorenal failure. 3 marks-any 6

Foetal complications are rare. Intrauterine growth restriction and foetal demise can happen in severe cases. 1 mark

IMPORTANT NOTE

The changes in blood chemistry with hyperemesis are as follows:

Haemoconcentration, leucocytosis, decrease in blood urea, hyponatremia, hypokalaemia, and hypochloraemic alkalosis, elevated liver enzymes and/or low TSH.

2. **A nulliparous woman at 30 weeks gestation presents at the labour ward with a BP of 180/110 mmHg and ++ protienuria. She has epigastric pain and right upper quadrant tenderness.**

a. **Describe your immediate management of the case.** (8 marks)

Admit her in high dependency unit (HDU) close to labour ward. 1 mark

Inform obstetric registrar and consultant along with anaesthesia registrar and senior labour room midwife about the case. 1 mark

Send baseline blood investigations which include a full blood counts, serum urea, creatinine, electrolytes, liver function tests and urinalysis. Repeat them every 12 to 24 hours as required. Peripheral blood smear to look for fragmented red blood cells, evidence of haemolysis and coagulation profile should be done. An electrocardiogram (EKG) should be recorded. 1 mark

Ultrasound to rule out other causes of upper abdominal pain. 1 mark

Foetal well-being should by assessed be continuous electronic foetal monitoring, measuring amniotic fluid index, and umbilical cord Doppler. 1 mark

All maternal observations should be recorded meticulously. These include; blood pressures every 15 min, continuous pulse oxymetry, urine output (Foley's catheterization) and hourly temperature. 1 mark

Commence antenatal steroids. 1 mark

Antihypertensives should be started (intravenous hydralazine or nifedepine) according to hospital protocols and availability. 1 mark

c. **After six hours, her proteinuria becomes +++, BP is 150/100 mmHg and liver enzymes are raised. How will you manage her now?**
 (8 marks)

HELLP syndrome is the most likely diagnosis and delivery is the only definitive treatment. Full blood counts, platelet count, liver function tests and LDH levels should be performed to confirm the diagnosis. Abnormal peripheral smear, serum bilirubine1.2 mg/dl, elevated liver enzymes–SGOT> 72IU/l, LDH> 600IU/l, low platelet count < 100,000 is diagnostic. 2 marks

Multidisciplinary treatment by involving surgeons (liver rupture), nephrologists (renal failure) and haematologists (coagulation defects) should be encouraged. 1 mark

Fluid balance should be strictly monitored and maintained at 85 ml/hr. Prefer colloids. 500 ml human albumin solution (HAS) should be administered prior to hydralazine, caesarean section, if urinary output is <100 ml in 4 hrs and before regional anaesthesia. 1 mark

CVP line should be inserted prior to giving HAS as risk of pulmonary oedema and fluid overload should be balanced with risk of acute renal failure due to hypovolaemia. 0.5 mark

Consider prophylactic magnesium sulphate according to hospital protocols. Serum magnesium levels should be considered if she has repeated seizures, absent deep tendon reflexes, SpO_2 < 95 percent (Respiratory rate >14) and oliguria is present. 1 mark

Coagulation defects should be corrected by infusions of fresh frozen plasma or platelet transfusions before delivery. 1 mark

If maternal and foetal condition permits and Bishop Score is favourable, induction may be tried. If platelet count is >100 × 10^9/l regional anaesthesia is safe. Likelihood of caesarean section remains high and delivery should take place in a hospital with good neonatal facilities. 1 mark

Ergometrine should be avoided in the postpartum period and intensive monitoring should continue for 72 hrs. Risk of recurrence is high-up to 40 percent in subsequent pregnancies. 0.5 mark

d. **You have informed the woman that an emergency section has to be performed to prevent deterioration in her condition. The couple wishes to know the implications for the baby. Since your paediatric colleague is not available at present; you have been asked to talk to the couple. What will you tell them?** **(4 marks)**

This baby has an 80 per cent chance of survival but she may require care in the NICU till an equivalent of 36 weeks of gestational age. 1 mark

Baby may have difficulty in maintaining its body temperature and have to be kept under warmers. Some babies (30% chance if less than 1.5 kg at birth) may start bleeding in their brain. This happens mostly during the first seven days because of which some babies may develop serious handicap later on in life. 1 mark

Pre-mature babies often have difficulty in breathing well and some may require support with ventilators in the nursery. Such babies often have to be fed with a tube; however expressed milk may be asked for by the paediatricians. 1 mark

Preterm babies remain at a higher risk of tummy upsets, infections, breathing problems and may require emergency surgery at times. Such babies usually require a lot of care in the first three months even when discharged well.   1 mark

IMPORTANT NOTE

Therapeutic levels of magnesium sulphate are 4-7 mEq/l.

Loss of patellar reflex occurs at 8-10 mEq/l.

Respiratory depression occurs at 10-12 mEq/l.

Respiratory arrest occurs at ≥12 mEq/l.

Cardiac arrest occurs at ≥25 mEq/l.

In 10 to 20 per cent patients of HELLP, BP may be normal to begin with.

Contraindications of administering magnesium sulphate are:

Myasthenia Gravis, hypocalcaemia, renal or heart disease, calcium channel blockers and known allergies.

3. **A 32-year-old parous woman is complainting of postcoital bleeding. She is anxious as she has heard that it could be a sign of cancer.**

a. **What are the possible causes of such bleeding in her?** **(4 marks)**

Common causes of postcoital bleeding at her age include infection, genital tract trauma, cervical or endometrial polyp, cervical ectropion and coincidental intermenstrual bleeding. Malignancy as a cause of bleeding is unlikely.   3 marks

Pregnancy related complications should be ruled out at the outset.   1 mark

b. **What relevant history would you enquire about?** **(6 marks)**

Detailed history should be elicited regarding the amount, frequency, duration of bleeding and its relation to intercourse.   1 mark

Menstrual history, intake of exogenous hormones, and history of trauma to genital tract are important.   2 marks

Excessive vaginal discharge, foul smell or any recent change in the discharge should be noted.   1 mark

Family history of cancers and the reason for her fear should be asked gently.
    1 mark

Possibility of bleeding disorder should be kept in mind if associated with other menstrual symptoms like intermittent intermenstrual bleeding or if she is on anticoagulant therapy.   1 mark

c. **Describe her management including the investigations.** **(10 marks)**

General physical examination (anaemia) and abdominal examination for abnormal masses should be done. Vulval inspection for signs of trauma and vulvitis, examination with cuscoes speculum (cervicitis, ectropion, and vaginal discharge) and bimanual examination of pelvis should be offered.   2 marks

Appropriate swabs for microscopy and cervical smear should be taken (if due) prior to bimanual examination.   1 mark

Perform a pregnancy test or serum b HCG if there is any possibility of pregnancy.
    1 mark

Transvaginal ultrasound for pelvic pathology and endometrial assessment for polyps. Endocervical polyps can be avulsed in outpatient setting. If post-coital bleeding continues than a formal hysteroscopic evaluation of endometrium during proliferative phase should be offered for endometrial sampling.   2 marks

Appropriate antimicrobial therapy and contact tracing should be offered if sexually transmitted diseases are a cause of cervicitis.   1 mark

Ectropion can cause PCB in 5 percent women. Superimposed infections are common. Cryotherapy or electrocauery is usually enough but occasionally ablative methods are required after treating infection and ensuring a normal smear.

2 marks

Referral for colposcopy and cervical biopsy should be done if there is suspicion of invasion or if the smear is abnormal.   1 mark

IMPORTANT NOTE

Triple swabs should be taken for ruling out sexually transmitted disease. One high vaginal swab for culture and two endocervical swabs for gonorrhoea culture and Chlamydia analysis.

4. **An 18-year-old woman complains of painful periods. She is not sexually active.**

   Discuss her management.   **(20 marks)**

She should have the physiological basis of pain explained sympathetically and provided with information booklets describing menstrual cycle and likely reasons of her symptom.   3 marks

Specific pathology is unlikely to be present in a young sexually inactive woman and this opportunity should be utilized to speak to the patient in the absence of her mother to explore family and social pressures.   3 marks

Pelvic examination is rarely helpful, ultrasound scanning is preferred if necessary. It reassures the woman and helps to exclude major pathology.   3 marks

Pain is related to prostaglandin release due to ovulation, therefore, non-steroidal antiinflammatory drugs started on the first day of period or pain, whichever is earlier, are the logical first line therapy.   2 marks

Combined oral contraceptives are also an effective treatment which may have additional benefits like reducing the flow and fulfilling the need for future contraception.   2 marks

Other options like luteal phase progestogens, danazol, calcium channel blockers and medicated IUCD may not be suitable for her but a trial of treatment for three months may be advisable after explaining the risks and benefits.   3 marks

If vomiting is present, non-oral treatment with antiemetics may be required.
                                                                        2 marks

Laparoscopy, to diagnose and treat underlying pathology, (endometriosis) is indicated only in resistant cases.   2 marks

IMPORTANT NOTE

During dysmenorrhoea plasma concentrations of vasopressin and myometrial concentrations of PGF 2α are high. While uterine blood flow decreases during pain.

Time allowed: 1.45 hours   *MM 80*

1. An 18-year-old woman reveals at her booking visit that she smokes 10 to 15 cigarettes in one day. She is currently 8 weeks pregnant.

    (10, 10 marks)
    a. What are the obstetric risks associated with her addiction?
    b. After hearing the risks she promises to give up her smoking habit. Describe the components of smoking cessation programme in UK.

2. Mrs Cathie has been admitted to the labour ward with spontaneous onset of labour at term. At 4 pm she was 5 cm dilated with head at –3 station. At 7 pm she was 6 cm dilated and leading part at –2 station.

    (9, 11 marks)
    a. Her partner appears concerned and wants to know if all is progressing well with the mother and baby. What is your management at this stage?
    b. At 1 am she was found to be pushing hard and partogram revealed that she has been fully dilated for more than two hours. You repeat a vaginal examination and find that the cervix is fully dilated and vertex is felt at plus 2 station. You decide to apply a ventouse as CTG has started to show non-reassuring foetal heart rate pattern. What will you keep in mind before proceeding?

3. You are an SpR_3 and while performing abdominal hysterectomy for endometriosis, a 3 cm long cut was seen on the bladder.
    a. Enumerate the further course of action.   (7 marks)
    b. Enumerate the precautions that you will take to minimize urinary morbidity during hysterectomy?   (13 marks)

4. A 35-year-old woman wishes to conceive and TVS done as part of investigations shows a cyst in the right ovary 5 × 4 cm in dimensions. Her pregnancy test is negative.
    Outline her management options.   (20 marks)

1. **An 18-year-old woman reveals at her booking visit that she smokes 10 to 15 cigarettes a day. She is currently 8 weeks pregnant.**

a. **What are the obstetric risks associated with her addiction?   (10 marks)**

Maternal risks are increased incidences of ectopic pregnancy, miscarriage, preterm delivery, and premature rupture of membranes.   2 marks

Smokers are up to three times more likely to experience placental abruption and/ or placenta praevia than non-smokers. Placenta praevia increases the risk of maternal bleeding and premature delivery of the foetus.   2 marks

Foetal growth restriction is more likely in foetuses exposed to parental smoking.
                                                                                                                                        1 mark

Preterm premature rupture of membranes leads to premature birth and increased risk of intrauterine infection and serious infection in the neonate.   2 marks

Reduction in breastfeeding is also associated with smoking.   1 mark

Low birth weight babies are at increased risk of illness in both the neonatal period and later life. Many studies have found a linear relationship between the numbers of cigarettes smoked in the third trimester of pregnancy and decreased foetal birth weight.   1 mark

Maternal smoking increases the risk of sudden infant death syndrome (sudden unexplained loss of life in the first year) by up to four-fold compared with controls.
                                                                                                                                        1 mark

b. **After hearing the risks she promises to give up her smoking habit. Describe the components of smoking cessation programme in UK.**
                                                                                                      (10 marks)

First-line intervention for pregnant women on initial diagnosis of nicotine dependence involves 'motivational' assessment, interviewing and individual or group-based 'talking' therapy offered in a stepwise fashion. One-to-one counselling should be provided by specially trained cessation advice nurses and/or group therapy clinics.   2 marks

Initial counselling may initially take the form of simply providing information regarding the availability of cessation services, the risks of smoking during pregnancy and the benefits of quitting. Counselling sessions are effective in pregnancy and lead to a reduction in the incidence of preterm birth and low birth weight. 2 marks

Second-stage intervention involves one-to-one or group counselling sessions, depending on the preferences and requirements of each individual. One-to-one counselling sessions are typically offered to pregnant women as a series of home visits or at a local primary care facility. Group therapy is typically offered at a primary care trust site as a specialist service to groups of between five and 25 individuals.   2 marks

The aim is to empower the individual to take responsibility for her own treatment and thereby increase the likelihood of sustainable change. A 'quit date' is then set and the number of cigarettes smoked reduced in the week prior to cessation. During this week, she is encouraged to complete a smoking diary, which is intended to reinforce behavioural change. After quitting, carbon monoxide tests may be carried out to gauge successful maintenance.   2 marks

Nicotine replacement therapy (NRT) can be considered in pregnant women under some circumstances.   1 mark

Pharmacological drugs such as bupropion and, varenicline, have proven effective in increasing cessation rates in the general population, but are contraindicated for use in pregnancy.   1 mark

IMPORTANT INFORMATION

The prevalence of smoking in general public in UK is coming down but smoking among pregnant women remains high (30% in new mothers). Smoking remains the single largest preventable cause of foetal and infant morbidity in the UK.

Nicotine crosses the placenta and causes a dose-related rise in maternal blood pressure and heart rate. Nicotine is metabolised 30 per cent more quickly in pregnancy.

Guidance from NICE recommends considering NRT for women who do not accept individual or group therapy and for those expressing a clear wish to receive it. They also recommend advising women to remove patches at night to avoid continuous foetal exposure to nicotine. The evidence for NRT efficacy and safety in pregnancy is, however, sparse and often contradictory. The risks of using NRT should be weighed against the harm potentially caused by continued smoking. NRT, if required should be used early in pregnancy with the aim of discontinuing use after 2 to 3 months.

Maternal smoking has been associated with an overall reduced incidence of pre-eclampsia because it may modulate factors involved in angiogenesis, endothelial function and the immune response.

There is a higher incidence of respiratory symptoms in children (including chronic cough, wheeze and breathlessness). Children may have higher likelihood of developmental/behavioural problems and obesity in their growing years.

2. **Mrs Cathie has been admitted to the labour ward with spontaneous onset of labour at term. At 4 pm she was 5 cm dilated with head at –3 station. At 7 pm she was 6 cm dilated and leading part at –2 station.**

a. **Her partner appears concerned and wants to know if all is progressing well with the mother and baby. What is your management at this stage?**
(9 marks)

When the rate of cervical dilatation is less than 1 cm/hr in the active phase, poor progress should be diagnosed.   1 mark

Her partogram should be reviewed to identify the pattern and duration of delay.
2 marks

Assess her hydration and nutrition levels. Start intravenous fluids and provide adequate analgesia.   1 mark

Rule out cephalopelvic disproportion, malposition (most likely occipito transverse or occipito posterior position) and malpresentation by accurate assessment prior to any intervention. Urine should be checked for ketones if she is exhausted.   2 marks

Start and check CTG. Check the frequency and duration of uterine contractions. Three contractions of moderate intensity, each lasting 40 to 45 sec, within ten minutes is optimum. Start oxytocin drip if required.   2 marks

Reassure and maintain watchful expectancy if maternal and foetal condition is satisfactory.   1 mark

b. **At 1 am she was found to be pushing hard and partogram revealed that she has been fully dilated for more than two hours. You repeat a vaginal examination and find that the cervix is fully dilated and vertex is felt at plus 2 station. You decide to apply a ventouse as CTG has started to show non-reassuring foetal heart rate pattern. What will you keep in mind before proceeding?**
(11 marks)

Recheck that no part or less than one fifths of foetal vertex is palpable abdominally.
2 marks

Membranes are ruptured and rotation of the head has been accurately ascertained. Pelvis should be adequate.   2 marks

Written informed consent with clear explanation should be taken from the mother.
1 mark

Her bladder should have been recently emptied or if indwelling catheter is in place, the balloon should be deflated. 1 mark

If epidural catheter has been sited, check for top up requirements or give adequate analgesia by local infiltration. 2 marks

Experienced staff should be available in labour ward and instruments should be checked before application. All possible aseptic precautions should be taken and a backup of forceps should be ready in case of failure. 1 mark

Anticipate shoulder dystocia and PPH (slow progress/ long labour) and be vigilant. 1 mark

Skilled neonatologist should preferably be present to take over the neonate.

1 mark

IMPORTANT NOTE

Inefficient uterine contractions are recognised as the commonest cause for poor progress.

Active management of labour comprises of amniotomy, early use of oxytocin, and continuous professional support to ensure optimal progress of labour and normal delivery. It decreases the risk of prolonged labour and associated morbidity of maternal infection, uterine rupture, post-partum haemorrhage and maternal death. The total duration of labour may be shortened by 60 to 120 min.

Active management is ineffective in reducing the rate of caesarean section or operative vaginal delivery. Early amniotomy leads to reduction in the duration of labour by 60 to 90 min, but may increase the risk of infection.

Optimal interval between dose increments of oxytocin is 30 min and dose should be started at 10 min/ml and titrated to achieve a contraction frequency of 4 in 10 min each lasting >40 seconds.

3. **You are an SpR$_3$ and while performing abdominal hysterectomy for endometriosis, a 3 cm long cut was seen on the bladder.**

a. **Enumerate the further course of action.** **(7 marks)**

Inform and call the gynaecological consultant for help. Summon urological colleagues. 1 mark

Visualise the anatomy and trace the ureters and ureteric openings. Complete the procedure in the mean time. Bladder should be closed in two overlapping layers with vicryl (3-0). 2 marks

A pelvic drain should be left *in situ*. Routine abdominal closure should be as routinely followed. She will require Foley's catheter *in situ* for 7 days. 1 mark

Postoperative antibiotics and thromboprophylaxis should be added according to her risk assessment. There is no real need for imaging unless there are concerns. 1 mark

Debrief the complication to the patient as soon as she is comfortable, acknowledging that the likelihood of such an incident happening is higher due to endometriosis. Appropriate risk management forms should be filled and case notes meticulously completed. 2 marks

b. **Enumerate the precautions that you will take to minimise urinary morbidity during hysterectomy?** **(13 marks)**

Appropriate preoperative assessment, investigations and exclusion of any pre-existent urinary dysfunction are important. Perform IVU (intravenous urogram) in case of high risk cases. 1 mark

Urine infection is commonly related to catheterisation and stasis of urine. Prophylactic antibiotics can reduce the infection rates. 1 mark

Risk of ureteric injury is higher in previous pelvic and uterine surgeries (LSCS), enlarged uterus, distorted pelvic anatomy, massive intraoperative haemorrhage, and endometriosis. High-index of suspicion should be kept in such cases. 1 mark

Laparoscopic procedures should be undertaken wherever possible, as the risk of injury to urinary passage is lower. 1 mark

Ureteric damage can be reduced by careful dissection, adequate exposure and good surgical technique, use of splints, help of urological colleagues and the judicious use of the subtotal operation. The bladder should be mobilised in a downward and outward direction so the ureters move away from the operative field. Blind clamping of bleeding vessels should be avoided in the vulnerable areas. Tissue haemostasis should be good so that formation of vault haematoma is avoided. 2 marks

Bladder damage can be avoided by careful dissection, an empty bladder, use of subtotal procedure, and the use of longer catheterisation with difficult dissections or presence of haematuria and the recognition and repair of injuries when they occur. 2 marks

Short-term voiding disorders are due to pain, immobility and excess IV fluids. Adequate analgesia, hydration and early ambulation should be encouraged.

1 mark

During laparoscopic surgery, short applications of diathermy should be encouraged to limit the thermal damage to urinary structures. 1 mark

If any ureteric injury is suspected, intraoperative ureteric catheterisation should be done and early urological assistance sought. Prompt and meticulous repair decreases the associated morbidity. Transurethral cystoscopy can visualise ureteric jets from both ureteric orifices. Its routine use should be promoted in complex cases. Use of wound drains should be encouraged. 2 marks

Seventy percent injuries are identified in the postoperative period. Vigilance should be maintained for symptoms like fever, haematuria, flank pain, abdominal distension, anuria and urinary leakage. 1 mark

IMPORTANT NOTE

Risk of ureteric damage is 1 in 500 for benign disease, and 1 in 100 for malignancy. Bladder damage occurs in 1 in 200 cases.

One can tackle such questions by dividing the precautions in preoperative, intra-operative and post-operative precautions. Also the question does not specify the type of hysterectomy, so think of all angles.

4. **A 35-year-old woman wishes to conceive and TVS done as part of investigations shows a cyst in the right ovary 5 × 4 cm in dimensions. Her pregnancy test is negative.**
   Outline her management options. (20 marks)

The majority of ovarian cysts in reproductive age group are functional and thus benign. None the less, every effort should be made to rule out malignancy. Detailed history should be elicited to exclude symptoms pertaining to other systems. Use of ovulation induction drugs like clomiphene citrate should be elicited. 2 marks

Investigations including the partner's semen analysis, tubal patency, day 21 serum progesterone and other routine investigations along with vaginal swabs should be checked as part of initial work-up for infertility. 3 marks

Detailed ultrasound appearance of the cyst should be sought. Increasing size, presence of septations, papillary formations, echogenic solid areas and free fluid in the pouch of Douglas may suggest ovarian malignancy. Risk of malignancy index (RMI) should be calculated combining her ultrasound findings, CA125 values and premenopausal status. 3 marks

If her RMI is less than 250, the risk of malignancy is considered low and she may be offered expectant management with a repeat scan 3 to 6 months later. Approximately 50 percent simple cysts resolve spontaneously. 2 mark

If the RMI is more than 250, further management should be planned with a gynaecological oncologist. 1 mark

In the absence of pain, hormonal suppression with combined oral contraceptives has no role. 1 mark

Cyst aspiration has a high chance of recurrence. 1 mark

Laparoscopic cyst removal may be offered as it carries a lower risk of postoperative adhesion formation that may compromise her future fertility, decreased blood loss, shorter hospital stay, more cosmetic results and lesser morbidity. She should be informed about the risk of laparoscopy, particularly bowel and major vessel injury and that she may require laparotomy, should any problems arise. 3 marks

Laparoscopic cystotomy and ablation or stripping of cyst wall may be offered for treatment of ovarian endometrioma. Bleeding, adhesion formation and loss of adjacent follicles are possible complications. 1 mark

Cystectomy (removal of intact cyst) may be offered for a dermoid cyst and if there is a possible chance of malignancy. 1 mark

Laparotomy may be required if there is a suspicion of malignancy or if she is unfit for laparoscopy because of obesity or extensive abdominal scarring. 2 marks

IMPORTANT NOTE

The risk of malignancy index (RMI) is calculated by 3 factors and scores are given for each of them:

RMI = U× M× CA125

U = 0 (for ultrasound score of zero)

U = 1 (for ultrasound score of 1)

U = 3 (for ultrasound score of 2-5)

Ultrasound scans are scored one point for each of the following characteristics:

Multilocular cyst, evidence of solid areas, evidence of metastasis, presence of ascitis, bilateral lesions.

M=1 for premenopausal and 3 for all postmenopausal women.

CA125 is the serum CA125 measurement in u/ml.

Time allowed: 1.45 hours   *MM 80*

1. A 24-year-old parous woman complains of painful intercourse 6 weeks after childbirth.   (5, 5, 10 marks)
   a. What could be the likely aetiology?
   b. What points in her history would you elicit to arrive at a diagnosis?
   c. How would you manage her?

2. A 20-year-old multigravida repeatedly presents at the day assessment unit with concerns about loss of foetal movements. She is currently 30 weeks in gestation. All the preliminary tests of foetal well-being are unremarkable. While you were reassuring her, she reveals that her husband is an alcoholic and abuses her.   (20 marks)
   Briefly outline your management plan.

3. A 26-year-old woman had secondary amenorrhoea for six months. During investigations her FSH was 52 IU/l and LH was 34 IU/l. Pregnancy test is negative and all other investigations are unremarkable. She wishes to conceive in the near future.   (15, 5 marks)
   a. What advice will you give regarding the diagnosis and management options?
   b. Enumerate the ethical issues regarding oocyte donation.

4. A 42-year-old healthy woman comes to you for contraceptive advice. How will you counsel her?   (20 marks)

1. A 24-year-old parous woman complains of painful intercourse 6 weeks after childbirth.

a. What could be the likely aetiology? (5 marks)

The aetiology could be related to delivery trauma, or due to breast-feeding dryness.

2 marks

At times cause could be pre-existing including physical problems like pelvic adhesions, PID, cervicitis, cystitis, scar tissue, and severe constipation, etc.

2 marks

Psychological causes and decreased libido could come to notice now. 1 mark

b. What points in her history would you elicit to arrive at a diagnosis? (5 marks)

Her own perspective of her problem, order of its development, social and family demands, privacy, financial support and availability of help at home, fear of pain and pregnancy, previous history of depression should be elicited. 2 marks

History of any hormonal contraceptives being used. 1 mark

Details of delivery, her experience during childbirth, breastfeeding and details of pain (on entry or deep) should be asked in a sensitive and non judgemental manner.

2 marks

c. How would you manage her? (10 marks)

She should be informed about decreased sexual interest after childbirth as >50 percent women report loss of sexual desire and discomfort on resuming sexual activity. 1 mark

Inspect the lower genital tract for any swelling, irritation, warts, varicosities, abrasions, poor anatomical alignment of perineal tears or episiotomy and scar tissue bands. Assisted vaginal delivery is more likely to be associated with perineal trauma. 1 mark

Gentle per speculum examination and swabs should be taken if infection is suspected. 1 mark

Examination should first include single finger insertion to rule out vaginismus and to avoid confusion with pelvic pain. Bimanual examination to elicit cervical excitation, and evidence of pelvic infection should be done with good lubrication.

1 mark

Pelvic ultrasound should be asked for if any pelvic pathology is suspected.

1 mark

Provide reassurance if due to tiredness or increased demands on her time. Water-based lubricant jelly should be prescribed to relieve vaginal dryness associated with breastfeeding.

1 mark

Modified Fenton's procedure and perineal refashioning may be offered at some stage for excessive scar tissue.

1 mark

Changing the positions of intercourse may be advisable for deep dyspareunia. Adequate contraception should be prescribed to dispel her fears of an unwanted pregnancy.

1 mark

If pre-existing or non-organic cause is found she should be referred to psychosexual therapist.

1 mark

Refractory cases may be referred to dedicated perineal care clinics with multidisciplinary input.

1 mark

2. **A 20-year-old multigravida repeatedly presents at the day assessment unit with concerns about loss of foetal movements. She is currently 30 weeks in gestation. All the preliminary tests of foetal well being are unremarkable. While you were reassuring her, she reveals that her husband is an alcoholic and abuses her.**
Briefly outline your management plan. (20 marks)

She should be handled sympathetically and calmly, with a non judgemental approach. 1 mark

Total confidentiality of the conversation should be assured. It is important to convey that she is being understood and taken seriously. 2 marks

Details about her family background, educational status, social and financial support should be enquired to give her practical suggestions. 2 marks

High risk behaviour should be identified by personal history of alcoholism, drug abuse, multiple sexual partners, treatment for depression and unwanted pregnancy. Any perceived threats to her or her children's life should be directly asked. 3 marks

Reassure her that it is not her fault that she is being abused and she must not allow the situation to continue. Domestic violence is on the increase and appropriate support is available. 2 marks

She should be encouraged to talk to someone in the family or friend whom she trusts. 2 marks

She can contact the domestic violence unit of local police for protection. Local women's aid groups can provide assistance with employment and temporary shelters. All possible help to get contact numbers should be provided. The police can be informed from the hospital on her behalf. In emergency situations short term hospital admission may be offered. She can prepare an escape plan with her children. 3 marks

Her complaints should be documented with her prior consent. General practitioner and area social worker should be involved. 2 marks

Follow up appointment should be arranged in the outpatient setting to reassure her about foetal well-being. Vigilance should be observed for obstetric complications like prematurity and abruption. 2 marks

The health worker should be notified of this history so that child abuse may be recognised early. 1 mark

IMPORTANT NOTE

50 percent men who abuse their wives, will also abuse their children.

3. **A 26-year-old woman had secondary amenorrhoea for six months. During investigations her FSH was 52 IU/l and LH was 34 IU/l. Pregnancy test is negative and all other investigations are unremarkable. She wishes to conceive in the near future.**

a. **What advice will you give regarding the diagnosis and management options?** **(15 marks)**

The investigations point towards a diagnosis of premature ovarian failure (POF).

1 mark

Menstrual history and other symptoms of menopause, e.g. hot flushes, night sweats, sleeping problems, vaginal dryness, and low energy drive or bladder control problems should be enquired and treatment offered accordingly.

2 marks

History of any other illness, chemotherapy, recent weight loss or surgery should be elicited. 1 mark

Hormonal analysis should be repeated after 4 to 6 weeks to confirm the diagnosis and estimate the ovarian reserve. 2 marks

She should be advised to conceive early. Only 6 to 8 out of a hundred women with POF will be able to conceive. 1 marks

Semen analysis of her partner and tubal patency should be checked. The couple should be advised to have regular intercourse after every 2 to 3 days. The couple will need referral to an ART centre. 2 marks

A lipid profile and bone densitometry may be advised. Ovarian biopsy and karyotyping are not indicated. 1 mark

She should be encouraged to eat a healthy diet and exercise regularly (aerobics and weight training) to decrease health risks of osteoporosis and heart disease.

1 mark

Advise her to quit smoking, as it can accelerate ovarian loss. Hormone replacement therapy should be started as the benefits of estrogen replacement outweigh the risks at her age and especially if she is experiencing symptoms. 2 marks

There is no way to restore follicular function in POF. Ovulation induction should be avoided as already the ovarian reserve is poor. Assessment of FSH and AMH (antimullerian hormone) may be done to assess ovarian reserve. 1 mark

Oocyte donation and adoption are other options. She should be given opportunities for bereavement counselling and put in touch with support groups.

1 mark

b. Enumerate the ethical issues regarding oocyte donation. **(5 marks)**

Donors have to undergo stimulation and younger women sometimes risk their own reproductive capabilities.

1 mark

Payment of oocyte donors turns oocytes into commodities, jeopardizes informed consent and may lead to exploitation of economically disadvantaged women.

2 marks

Risk of transmission of communicable diseases including HIV, Hepatitis B should be minimized by appropriate screening tests of both the donor and recipient.

1 mark

Relatives acting as oocyte donors may disturb the social fabric of society.

1 mark

IMPORTANT NOTE

In this condition, there is a premature loss of ovarian function; usually before 40 years, either through an accelerated loss or dysfunction of eggs. The reason could vary from a chromosomal or enzymatic defect to viral infection and autoimmune diseases. Sometimes it may not be possible to pinpoint a cause. It should be emphasized that stress is not a cause of POF and she is not responsible for it. It may be hereditary in 5 percent women.

Elevated FSH values above 40 iu/l repeated twice over 4 to 6 weeks suggest POF in a woman less than 40 years. The value fluctuate with time and higher the FSH levels, lower is the ovarian reserve and lower are a woman's chances to conceive. HRT with estrogens will decrease FSH values but will not increase the follicular reserve or function.

4. A 42-year-old healthy woman comes to you for contraceptive advice. How will you counsel her? **(20 marks)**

She should be informed that although a natural decline in fertility occurs from the age of 37 years, regular ovulation still occurs and effective contraception is required to prevent unplanned pregnancy. 2 marks

The contraceptive choice for her may be influenced by many factors—frequency of intercourse, natural decline in fertility, sexual function, the wish for non-contraceptive benefits, menstrual dysfunction, concurrent medical conditions and her smoking habits. 2 marks

A clinical history, including sexual history should be taken to assess the contraceptive options, taking account of cardiovascular and cerebrovascular disease and neoplasia, which increase with age. 1 mark

No contraceptive is contraindicated by age alone. She should be informed about the risks and non-contraceptive benefits of all contraceptive methods and allowed to make an informed decision. 2 marks

She can use combined hormonal contraception including the pills (COC) unless there are co-existing diseases or risk factors. Monophasic pills with less than 30 µg ethinylestradiol and low dose of norethisterone or levonorgestrel should be preferred as the first line option. COC's may increase her bone mineral density, reduce incidence of hip fractures, cause a 50 percent reduction in risk of ovarian, endometrial cancer and colorectal cancer, decrease her incidence of benign breast disease, menstrual bleeding, pain and hot flushes. There may be a reduction in incidence of functional ovarian cysts, benign ovarian tumors, acne and rheumatoid arthritis. No causal association between COC use and weight gain has been found. 4 marks

There is no apparent increase in risk of cardiovascular disease or stroke with progesterone only contraceptives. Long acting reversible contraceptives like LNG-IUS (Mirena) and implants are safe to use even if she had a previous history of ischemic heart disease or VTE. There is no significant increase in breast cancer risk. However, there may be a slight decrease in BMD and irregular bleeding associated with POC use. 3 marks

Information about permanent methods, i.e. vasectomy and tubal occlusion with their advantages, disadvantages and relative failures should also be discussed. 1 mark

She may use barrier methods without spermicidal lubricant, which also help to prevent STI's. 1 mark

Copper intrauterine devices are safe to use. An endocervical swab to detect *Chlamydia* and gonorrhea should be offered and risk of menstrual abnormalities in the first few months explained. Once inserted, it can be left *in situ* until the menopause.   2 marks

Natural family planning methods like withdrawal are not reliable and hence not recommended.   1 mark

She should continue contraception until post-menopause is confirmed (After one year of amenorrhoea) or at 52 years.   1 mark

IMPORTANT NOTE

Average age of peri-menopause in UK is 46 years and lasts for approximately 5 years. Average age of menopause is 50.7 years.

Time allowed: 1.45 hours   *MM 80*

1. A primigravida has been referred to you at 41 completed weeks by the GP.   (10, 3, 7 marks)
   a. She wishes to discuss the management options with you. Which options would you counsel her for?
   b. She is keen for a totally natural labour and declines induction at present. How will you monitor her?
   c. Three days later; after the ultrasound, she changes her mind and agrees for induction of labour. Briefly outline the procedure that will be followed.

2. A primigravida with 32 weeks pregnancy presents at the labour ward with high-grade fever, headache and malaise. She is pale, icteric and has enlarged liver and spleen. Other systemic examination is unremarkable. She has just returned from a family vacation in Africa.   (3, 5, 3, 9 marks)
   a. Which relevant findings on history and examination would help you make a diagnosis?
   b. Describe the relevant investigations.
   c. Enumerate the complications arising out of this condition.
   d. Describe her relevant management.

3. You were performing diagnostic laparoscopy on a 37-year-old infertile woman, when after entry, you noticed fecal matter inside the peritoneal cavity.   (9, 5, 6 marks)
   a. Describe your immediate course of actions.
   b. On laparotomy you realise that there is a one-cm-long rent in the colon. How will you close the wound?
   c. Describe the relevant post-operative care for this patient.

4. A young college student has had an unprotected intercourse during a Saturday night party. She comes to you on Monday morning requesting post-coital contraception to avoid getting pregnant.   (6, 14)
   a. What are the issues involved?
   b. What are the options for emergency contraception for her?

1. A primigravida has been referred to you at 41 completed weeks by the GP.

a. She wishes to discuss the management options with you. Which options would you counsel her for? **(10 marks)**

The management options are active induction of labour after 41 weeks or expectant management with regular foetal monitoring. 2 marks

Before choosing any option accurate dating should be established, ideally from first trimester ultrasound. She should be re-evaluated for any foetal or maternal risk factors necessitating urgent intervention. 2 marks

She should be counselled for relative risks and benefits of induction vs. expectant management. Her wishes, cervical scoring and availability of ante-partum testing facilities should be taken into consideration when management is planned.
2 marks

Beyond 41 weeks, the incidence of meconium staining of amniotic fluid, need for intrapartum foetal blood sampling, shoulder dystocia, foetal hypoxia and foetal death increase due to uteroplacental insufficiency. There are increased rates of neonatal seizure and death. Delivery at 42 weeks was associated with doubling of perinatal mortality rate compared with delivery at 39 to 41 weeks. 2 marks

There are increased risks of instrumental and operative delivery and haemorrhage in her with an overall increase in maternal mortality. Her anxiety may increase as she passes her estimated date of delivery. 1 mark

To decrease the increase risk of maternal and foetal morbidity, she should be offered admission for induction of labour beyond 41 weeks. 1 mark

b. She is keen for a totally natural labour and declines induction at present. How will you monitor her? **(3 marks)**

From 42 weeks, she should be offered increased antenatal monitoring consisting of at least twice weekly cardio-tocography and ultrasound estimations of maximum amniotic fluid pool depth. 2 marks

She should be informed that monitoring may not be effective in reducing the incidence of 'post mature' foetal deaths. 1 mark

c. Three days later; after the ultrasound, she changes her mind and agrees for induction of labour. Briefly outline the procedure that will be followed. **(7 marks)**

Prior to formal induction of labour she should be offered a vaginal examination for membrane sweep. Nipple stimulation or regular coitus is an alternative if examination is refused. 2 marks

Labour can be induced with prostaglandin E2 pessaries (3 mg), followed if necessary by oxytocin or misoprostol and artificial rupture of membranes.

2 marks

Labour should be monitored by continuous foetal heart rate monitoring. Amnioinfusion may be considered for meconium staining of liquor or FHR abnormalities associated with oligohydramnios.   2 marks

In the presence of coexisting medical or obstetrical complicating factors, caesarean section should be performed.   1 mark

IMPORTANT NOTE

Term traditionally means period of gestation from 37 weeks plus 6 days till 40 weeks +7 days (37 completed weeks to 41 weeks).

2. **A primigravida with 32 weeks pregnancy presents at the labour ward with high grade fever, headache and malaise. She is pale, icteric and has enlarged liver and spleen. Other systemic examination is unremarkable. She has just returned from a family vacation in Africa.**

a. **Which relevant findings on history and examination would help you to make a diagnosis?** (3 marks)

There should be a high index of suspicion for malaria on account of her travel history. 1 mark

The predominant symptoms are fever, rigors, nausea, abdominal pain, body ache and headache. 1 mark

Look for pallor, jaundice, moderate and tender hepatosplenomegaly on examination. 1 mark

b. **Describe the relevant investigations.** (5 marks)

Diagnosis is made by detection of parasites on peripheral blood smear. 1 mark

Thick smear is required for diagnosis and thin film for identification of species. A rapid dipstick immunological test is reserved for *P. falciparum* infection. 2 marks

Samples should be withdrawn between 4 to 6 hours after spike of temperature due to increased parasitemia at that time. Serial samples may be required for diagnosis. Parasites in >2 per cent red cells indicate severe infection. 1 mark

Full blood counts, haematocrit, platelet count, renal functions, liver enzymes and blood sugar should be checked once and then periodically. HIV testing should be offered. 1 mark

c. **Enumerate the complications arising out of this condition.** (3 marks)

Maternal complications include hypoglycaemia, severe anaemia, pulmonary oedema, acute renal failure, hepatitis, hyperpyrexia, cerebral malaria, haemorrhagic and septicaemic shock. 1 mark

There are higher chances of intrauterine foetal hyperpyrexia causing preterm labour, foetal acidosis and still births. 1 mark

1 per cent babies are born with congenital malaria and may have fever, irritability, feeding problems, anaemia, jaundice and hepatosplenomegaly. 1 mark

d. **Describe her relevant management.** (9 marks)

Supportive management involves appropriate airway protection, fluid replacement while watching for development of pulmonary oedema and hypoglycaemia. 1 mark

Fever should be tackled by adequate exposure, fans, tepid sponging, and paracetamol. 1 mark

Screen her for anaemia and give blood transfusions if required. Dialysis for renal failure should be available. 1 mark

Cerebral malaria is a medical emergency with 15 to 20 per cent mortality rates. Intensive care treatment and multidisciplinary approach is essential. I.V. antibiotics along with antimalarials should be given due to increased susceptibility of pneumococcal and gram-negative septicaemia. 1 mark

Foetal surveillance with antenatal corticosteroids, daily nonstress test and serial ultrasounds should be maintained. Cord blood smear should be taken after delivery to rule out congenital malaria. 1 mark

Treatment should be by most effective antimalarial drug available. Choice of drug depends on pattern of local drug resistance, disease severity, drug safety and availability. Falciparum malaria may be multi-drug resistant. 1 mark

Chloroquine is the drug of choice for *P. vivax, P. malariae and P. ovale*. Primaquine is contraindicated in pregnancy but is safe during breastfeeding. Safety of newer drugs, i.e. halofentrine, lumefantrine, atovaqunone has not been established in pregnancy. 1 mark

Intravenous artesunate or quinine should be used for complicated *P. falciparum* infection. Both are safe for use in pregnancy. Quinine or clindamycin should be used for treatment of uncomplicated *P. falciparum* infection. 1 mark

Indications for urgent delivery are mainly acute foetal distress. Paediatrician should be present at the time of delivery and congenital malaria ruled out. 1 mark

IMPORTANT NOTE

Malaria spreads by bite of female anopheles mosquitoes, rarely by blood transfusion, vertical transmission and needle stick injury.

Paroxysms of fever are typical of the species;

Every 48 hours – P. vivax and P. ovale.

36 to 48 hours – P. falciparum.

72 hours – P. malariae.

80 per cent of global malaria burden occurs in Sub-Saharan Africa.

3. **You were performing diagnostic laparoscopy on a 37-year-old infertile woman when after entry, you noticed foecal matter inside the peritoneal cavity.**

a. **Describe your immediate course of actions.** **(9 marks)**

Inform the anaesthetist about the complication. 1 mark

Inform the consultant gynaecologist on call and ask one of the theatre staff to contact a general surgeon to request their assistance and advice. 2 marks

Request the anaesthetist to insert a nasogastric tube and commence intravenous antibiotics, e.g. Augmentin/Metronidazole and Cefuroxime. 2 marks

Proceed laparoscopically to identify the injury with the assistance of a general laparoscopic surgeon if the expertise for intra-abdominal suturing exists. If the culprit is the verress needle, closure of the perforation with suction of the foecal matter and generous peritoneal toilet may be sufficient. 2 marks

If the injury is due to a trocar or there is difficulty in delineating the site of injury, open the abdominal cavity by midline incision and define the extent of injury by careful inspection. 1 mark

Prevent spread of foeces throughout the peritoneal cavity by local packing. 1 mark

b. **On laparotomy you realize that there is a one cm long rent in the colon. How will you close the wound?** **(5 marks)**

Suture the defect with two layers of absorbable suture material with inversion of the colonic mucosa. 1 mark

Consider a defunctioning colostomy and a corrugated drain, as this perforated bowel may not have been prepared. 2 marks

The wound should be sutured with non-absorbable suture material to the sheath, and the skin should be sutured with interrupted nylon or prolene sutures because of the risk of wound infection. 2 marks

b. **Describe the relevant post-operative care for this patient.** **(6 marks)**

Post-operatively, continue intravenous fluids and keep nasograstric tube *in situ*. 1 mark

Broad spectrum antibiotics and adequate thromboprophylaxis should be administered. 2 marks

Debrief the patient as soon as she is comfortable, explaining the situation and why the colostomy was needed to enable successful bowel healing and that the colostomy will be closed in 6 to 12 weeks time. 2 marks

Complete the documentation and fill-up risk assessment forms. 1 mark

4. **A young college student has had an unprotected intercourse during a Saturday night party. She comes to you on Monday morning requesting post-coital contraception to avoid getting pregnant.**

a. **What are the issues involved?** (6 marks)

Accurate menstrual and sexual history, number and timing of intercourse should be elicited to assess her risk of pregnancy but there is no time in the menstrual cycle when there is zero risk of pregnancy following unprotected intercourse (UPSI).
2 marks

In addition to the risk of conception there may be a risk of sexually transmitted infection and HIV if the partner's background is not known. 1 mark

She should be given verbal and written information regarding the failure rates of oral and intra-uterine emergency contraception (EC) and allowed to make an informed decision. 1 mark

Advice on future contraception and follow-up to exclude pregnancy is essential. Information leaflets for the same should be provided. 2 marks

b. **What are the options for emergency contraception for her?** (14 marks)

She should be offered a single dose of levonorgestral 1.5 mg as soon as possible and within 72 hours of UPSI. This offers a success rate of eighty four out of 100.
2 marks

In case she misses the 72 hour deadline, she may take it anytime till 120 hours after UPSI for reducing the pregnancy chances (success rate 60%). If she vomits within 2 hours of taking LNG, she should return as soon as possible for a repeat dose. 3 marks

Oral mifepristone in a single dose has been found to be effective but is not yet licensed for EC use. It is more likely to act as an abortifacient as well by disturbing the implantation. 1 mark

The insertion of an appropriate copper bearing IUCD, up to 5 days after the first episode of UPSI, is the most effective option with an expected success rate of nearly 100 per cent. It can either be removed after the next period or left *in situ* as a longer term method of contraception. Risk of sexually transmitted infections, young age and nulliparity are not contraindications to IUD use. 3 marks

Chlamydia screening should be offered and prophylactic antibiotics considered prior to insertion of IUCD. Follow-up visits should be arranged to exclude infection, perforation or expulsion. 2 marks

She may experience bleeding disturbances in her cycle after taking LNG and over half of all women have their periods coming before or after the expected time. Risk of ectopic pregnancy is small but she must report to the hospital for any cycle irregularity and delay. She should use effective contraception or abstinence for the rest of the cycle.   3 marks

IMPORTANT NOTE

LNG EC is effective primarily by inhibiting ovulation. If given prior to LH surge, it inhibits ovulation for 5 to 7 days. It will not affect existing pregnancy and till now is not known to have any adverse effects on foetus.

Time allowed: 1.45 hours   *MM 80*

1. You are asked to see a 15-year-old girl in the early weeks of pregnancy.
   (8, 12 marks)
   a. How does antenatal care in a young teenager differ due to her age?
   b. What are the relevant issues for managing a young pregnant woman?

2. A 34-year-old woman on thyroxine supplements for hypothyroidism comes to you for advice. She is asymptomatic at present and wishes to start her family. (12, 8 marks)
   a. How will you counsel her?
   b. She comes to you six months later with a 10 weeks pregnancy. How will you manage the rest of her pregnancy?

3. An 18-year-old woman with a BMI of 34 has been found to have a picture consistent with polycystic ovaries on ultrasound done as a part of investigations for irregular periods. (7, 7, 6 marks)
   a. How will you arrive at a diagnosis?
   b. How will you manage her?
   c. What are the long-term consequences for her due to this condition?

4. A 38-year-old parous woman has been experiencing a dull ache in her lower abdomen for many months with occasional exacerbations of pain. All preliminary investigations have been unremarkable. (9, 11 marks)
   a. Discuss the relevant history, examination and investigations that are needed for her case.
   b. A diagnosis consistent with adenomyosis has been made and now she wishes hysterectomy. What are the issues involved in taking the consent for the procedure?

1. **You are asked to see a 15-year-old girl in the early weeks of pregnancy.**

a. **How does antenatal care in a young teenager differ due to her age?**
(8 marks)

Majority of teenage pregnancies may be unwanted and unplanned. They usually have poor compliance with antenatal care and should be encouraged for regular attendance.   2 marks

Healthy eating habits should be stressed to avoid risk of nutritional deficiencies. Adequate supplements should be prescribed.   1 mark

Early pregnancy ultrasound scan should be done to confirm gestational age.
1 mark

Associated cigarette smoking, alcohol consumption and recreational drug use are common amongst pregnant adolescents. A specific risk and need analysis should be done early and interventional strategies sought.   2 marks

Risk of sexually transmitted diseases is higher as she may not be in a stable relationship. If positive, referral to genitourinary clinics and appropriate contact tracing should be advised. Tests for *Chlamydia*, HIV, and syphilis should be offered.
2 marks

b. **What are the relevant issues for managing a young pregnant woman?**
(12 marks)

Antepartum: She should be handled sympathetically and enquiries should be made about perceived social isolation and financial difficulties.   1 mark

Multidisciplinary team with a social worker, family doctor and a dedicated midwife should be involved in her care. Special care should be given to allow her to continue her education at school or by a home tutor and emphasise compliance. 2 marks

Medical risks include anaemia, urinary tract infection, hypertension, and preterm labour.   1 mark

Information leaflets about pregnancy, breastfeeding, delivery and childrearing should be provided.   1 mark

She should be encouraged to involve and confide in family members or friends whom she trusts.   1 mark

Intrapartum: They have higher analgesia requirement and operative assistance during labour.   1 mark

Shoulder dystocia and obstructed labour is a possibility, keeping the small pelvis in mind.   1 mark

Involvement of partner or family members for psychological support during labour should be promoted. If her physical development is still immature, she should be referred to an equipped unit for delivery. 1 mark

Post-partum: There is a shorter interval to next pregnancy, low birth weight babies and sudden infant death syndrome. 1 mark

After delivery, feeding practises, infant safety, (child protection issues, possible abuse) social and financial concerns should be discussed openly. 1 mark

Effective contraception should be advised and adequate supplies issued, if required. Use of condoms should be encouraged to prevent sexually transmitted diseases. 1 mark

2. **A 34-year-old woman on thyroxine supplements for hypothyroidism comes to you for advice. She is asymptomatic at present and wishes to start her family.**

   How will you counsel her? **(12 marks)**

Enquiries regarding duration, dosage, type of supplement being taken and any pertinent symptoms should be made.   2 marks

Baseline thyroid functions and drug levels should be measured and pregnancy deferred untill medical optimisation has been achieved.   1 mark

General advice regarding rubella status, cigarette smoking, cervical screening and folic acid supplementation should be given.   1 mark

If she is already on adequate replacement therapy, reassurance should be offered, as maternal and foetal outcome is usually good and unaffected by the hypothyroidism.   1 mark

Untreated hypothyroidism may be associated with infertility, an increased rate of miscarriage, anaemia, pre-eclampsia, low birth weight infants, prematurity, still birth and foetal loss. Even subclinical hypothyroidism may be associated with reduced intelligence quotient and neurodevelopmental delay in the offspring. Severe deficiency may cause permanent brain damage and neurological deficiencies in the child.   3 marks

Very little thyroxine crosses the placenta and the foetus is not at risk of thyrotoxicosis from maternal thyroxine replacement therapy. Neonatal hypothyroidism may rarely result from transplacental passage of TSH receptor blocking antibodies.   2 marks

Pregnancy itself has no effect on disease progression. Early pregnancy is characterized by relative hyperthyroidism whereas there is a small decline in T_3 and T_4 levels in the second and third trimesters but all parameters remain within the normal range. If she is euthyroid at the beginning of pregnancy, usually no further increments in her thyroxine doses are required during pregnancy or in the puerperium.   2 marks

b. **She comes to you six months later with a 10 weeks pregnancy. How will you manage the rest of her pregnancy?** **(8 marks)**

Free T_4 (low), TSH (high), thyroid auto antibodies (may be present), complete blood counts, (normocytic anaemia), lipid profile (hyperlipidemia), liver function (deranged) and any specific investigations regarding the cause of hypothyroidism may be done at booking visit.   2 marks

Hypothyroidism may be associated with other autoimmune disorders like insulin dependent diabetes mellitus, pernicious anaemia and vitiligo. Search and appropriate investigations to rule out the same should be carried out. 1 mark

Thyroid functions should be done during the first trimester and at least once during each trimester to ensure adequate replacement. Following any adjustment in thyroxine dose, thyroid function should be checked after 4 to 6 weeks. Any increments in doses should be made cautiously in case of heart disease. 2 marks

Drugs like iron supplements and antacids containing aluminium hydroxide interfere with thyroxine absorption and should be taken at different times. 1 mark

No specific plans are needed for labour or delivery if she is adequately controlled. 1 mark

One in ten women will have residual postpartum dysfunction with an initial hyperthyroidism which may last for 2 to 3 months postpartum, followed by hypothyroidism. Management during initial puerperium should be symptomatic and 4 weekly assessment of antimicrosomal antibody titers. 1 mark

IMPORTANT NOTE

The commonest causes of hypothyroidism in women are iodine deficiency and autoimmune thyroiditis.

Placenta is freely permeable to TRH, TSH auto antibodies and iodine, not to TSH and thyroxine. Isolated thyroid nodules detected in pregnancy are likely to be malignant as most of the pregnancy related enlargement is diffused.

Foetus is dependent on maternal thyroid hormone until autonomous foetal thyroid function begins at 12 weeks. Thyroxine is important for foetal brain development, myelination and Purkinje cell function.

3. **An 18-year-old woman with a BMI of 34 has been found to have a picture consistent with polycystic ovaries on ultrasound done as a part of investigations for irregular periods.**

a. **How will you arrive at a diagnosis?** **(7 marks)**

One in four women will show ultrasound appearance of polycystic ovaries. History of hyperandrogenic symptoms like acne, hirsutism, hair loss etc. should be identified. 2 marks

Polycystic ovarian syndrome is diagnosed when 2 out of 3 criteria are fulfilled: Presence of oligo- and/or anovulation, hyperandrogenism and ultrasound evidence of polycystic ovaries. 1 mark

The recommended baseline screening tests are thyroid function tests, a serum prolactin and a free androgen index (total testosterone divided by sex hormone binding globulin (SHBG) x 100 to give a calculated free testosterone level). Urine pregnancy test should be done if required. 2 marks

In cases of clinical evidence of hyperandrogenism and total testosterone greater than 5 nmol/l,17-hydroxyprogesterone should be sampled and an androgen-secreting tumour should be excluded. 1 mark

If there is a clinical suspicion of Cushing's syndrome, this should be investigated according to local practice. 1 mark

b. **How will you manage her?** **(7 marks)**

The correction of obesity by diet and exercise offers the best chance of minimising the sequelae of PCOS. It may be more difficult for her to reduce weight and oral metformin may be tried to improve insulin resistance. In women unable to tolerate metformin, pioglitazone and inositol products may be tried. 2 marks

Initially, hirsutism should be managed by cosmetic methods. Finasteride and/or spironolactone may be required in severe cases but the effect of these preparations take a long time to show results. 2 marks

The use of combined pills will regulate her menstrual cycle and prevent endometrial hyperplasia. Drosperinone or cyproterone acetate pills are preferred due to their anti-mineralocorticoid and anti-androgenic effects. 2 marks

Ovarian electrocautery may help to reduce persistent anovulation once her BMI has been corrected. 1 mark

c. What are the long-term consequences for her due to this condition?
(6 marks)

Infertility and related psychological consequences may occur if her anovulation is resistant.   1 mark

Long-term consequences are an increased risk of developing type II diabetes mellitus, gestational diabetes, dyslipidemia and cardiovascular disease.   2 marks

Endometrial hyperplasia and later carcinoma is a possibility especially if she does not have regular bleeds. No increase in breast cancer and ovarian cancer risk has been found.   2 marks

Risk of sleep apnoea with resultant snoring and day time somnolence is increased depending upon her BMI and fat.   1 mark

IMPORTANT NOTE

The diagnosis of PCOS comprises of fulfilling two out of three criteria below:
1. *Polycystic ovaries (either 12 or more peripheral follicles or increased ovarian volume, 10 cm^3*
2. *Oligo or anovulation*
3. *Clinical and/or biochemical signs of hyperandrogenism.*

A raised luteinizing hormone/follicle stimulating hormone ratio is no longer a diagnostic criterion for PCOS owing to its inconsistency.

The diagnosis of PCOS can only be made when other aetiologies including thyroid dysfunction, hyperprolactinemia, androgen secreting tumours and cushing's syndrome have been excluded.

Women presenting with PCOS, especially if they are obese (body mass index greater than 30), have a strong family history of type 2 diabetes or are over the age of 40 years are at increased risk of type 2diabetes and should be offered a glucose tolerance test.

Sleep apnoea is an independent cardiovascular risk factor and has been found to be more common in PCOS. The difference in prevalence of sleep apnoea between PCOS and controls remained significant even when controlled for BMI. The strongest predictors for sleep apnoea were fasting plasma insulin levels and glucose-to-insulin ratios.

There is no association of PCOS with breast or ovarian cancer and no additional surveillance is required.

4. **A 38-year-old parous woman has been experiencing a dull ache in her lower abdomen for many months with occasional exacerbations of pain. All preliminary investigations have been unremarkable.**

a. **Discuss the relevant history, examination and investigations that are needed for her case.** **(9 marks)**

History should be detailed and include relationship to periods, pain with coitus, exacerbating factors, dietary history, sexual history, drug history (codeine), direct questions on gastrointestinal systems, diet and past psychological problems and abuse. 2 marks

The possibility of non-gynecological problems include functional and inflammatory bowel conditions (irritable bowel syndrome, Crohn's disease or ulcerative colitis), pelvic inflammatory disease, endometriosis, adnexal neoplasm and pelvic congestion syndrome should be considered. 1 mark

Examination includes general physical and bimanual vaginal examination. These may reveal pelvic masses, cervical fullness and fixed retroversion. Endocervical swabs should be taken for microbiology to exclude Chlamydia or other infections. 2 marks

Investigations should be directed by the history. Midstream urinalysis, renal ultrasound and bowel studies may be necessary. Abdominal and transvaginal ultrasound is reassuring to the women and occasionally reveal pathology not noted on clinical examination. 2 marks

Diagnostic laparoscopy may be required if no other cause is identifiable but it carries risk and may lead to confounding diagnosis and erroneous treatment. (For example, minimal endometriosis). 2 marks

b. **The diagnosis is consistent with adenomyosis and she now wishes hysterectomy. What are the issues involved in taking the consent for the procedure.** **(11 marks)**

She should be clearly informed about the name, nature of surgery and the reason of performing it. This will stop her periods and symptoms not related to uterus will not be affected. 1 mark

Other medical, less invasive procedures like insertion of LNG-IUS should have already been discussed and she should clearly have shown a disinclination to use them. 1 mark

She should be made aware of the type of anaesthesia planned and she may discuss it with the anaesthetist prior to surgery. 1 mark

The advantages and disadvantages of concomitant oophorectomy should be clearly discussed, keeping in mind her age, pathology, family history and possibility of having to take HRT.   2 marks

She should be informed of the serious and frequently occurring risks of the procedure. Risk of complications are higher if she is obese, has had previous surgery or pre-existing medical conditions.   1 mark

The frequent side-effects include wound infection, bruising, frequency of micturition, delayed wound healing, keloid formation and early menopause.
                                                                                1 mark

Risk of damage to bladder, bowel, and blood vessels should be explained and the repair of same may be required during the surgery.   1 mark

One in a 100 women requires blood transfusion and consent of the same should be taken separately, especially if she is a Jehovah's witness. There is a small risk of pelvic abscess, infection, VTE, return to theater in case of complications. All operations carry a risk of death which is 1 in 4000.   2 marks

She should be told that post-operatively she may have TED stockings, intravenous line, urinary catheter and a possible enema.   1 mark

IMPORTANT NOTE

Oophorectomy without consent may constitute assault.

Conditions where oophorectomy is beneficial, are a positive family history of breast or ovarian cancers, abnormal looking ovaries pre operatively, or there is uncontrolled bleeding from the site and oophorectomy can control this bleeding. Some benign diseases may be better treated by including oophorectomy, e.g. endometriosis, PID, unexpected pathology found at surgery and where there are unwanted ovarian endocrine effects, e.g. PMS, hirsutism, mastalgia.

The advantages of oophorectomy relate to the prevention of ovarian cancer and avoidance of a possible future surgery for subsequently developing ovarian pathology.

The disadvantages of oophorectomy relate to the loss of libido, which may be difficult or impossible to treat and the longer is the use of HRT, the greater is the increased risk of breast cancer – although this risk may be less with the use of SERMs.

Time allowed: 1.45 hours   *MM 80*

1. There has been an outbreak of B-19 parvovirus infection in a nursery school and a school teacher at 13 weeks gestation is worried about the implications on her pregnancy.   **(14, 6 marks)**
   a. What are the issues involved?
   b. What are the complications due to Parvovirus?

2. A 32-year-old multigravida woman has had a clot in her leg two years back. She is currently 8 weeks pregnant.   **(7, 13 marks)**
   a. What are the risk factors for developing thromboembolism in a pregnant woman?
   b. How will this information change your management of the remainder of her pregnancy?

3. A 49-year-old woman with heavy periods has an endometrial biopsy as part of investigations. Histopathology shows endometrial hyperplasia. Justify her further investigations and management.   **(20 marks)**

4. A couple approaches you for tubal ligation as they have completed their family. Outline the briefs of your counselling.   **(20 marks)**

1. **There has been an outbreak of B-19 parvovirus infection in a nursery school and a school teacher at 13 weeks gestation is worried about the implications on her pregnancy.**

a. **What are the issues involved?**   (14 marks)

In school outbreaks, one-thirds of susceptible staff contracts B-19 infection. Vertical transmission occurs in 30 percent of these maternal infections and may result in severe foetal infections. Being in constant touch with small children at workplace or home increases her susceptibility to acquire B-19 infection.   2 marks

Determine her serostatus for B-19 parvovirus by ELISA and western blot. In the presence of IgG and absence of IgM, she should be reassured as she is immune to infection. 50 per cent of adults are immune.   2 marks

If she is susceptible (IgG negative, IgM negative), but not yet infected, consideration may be given to exclude her from classrooms till 20 weeks of gestation. Repeat testing 3 weeks later.   2 marks

If maternal infection is confirmed (IgM positive), serial ultrasound scans should be done weekly for the next 8 to 10 weeks to detect foetal hydrops at the earliest. Infection in pregnancy is not an indication for therapeutic termination.   2 marks

Referral to a tertiary foetal medicine unit should be done once foetal hydrops is diagnosed. Foetal blood sample should be taken by Percutaneous umbilical blood sampling (PUBS) to assess the degree of anaemia. PUBS carries a complication rate of 1 per cent.   2 marks

If foetal anaemia is severe, intrauterine blood transfusions and early delivery after a course of steroids is advised.   2 marks

Conservative management and reassessment is appropriate if anaemia is mild and foetal reticulocyte count is high. Hydrops due to B-19 infection is caused due to foetal anaemia and resolves spontaneously in one-third-cases.   2 marks

b. **What are the complications due to parvovirus?**   (6 marks)

25 per cent of all infections in adults are asymptomatic.   1 mark

Fever, rash, malaise, arthralgia, and haemolytic anaemia may be the presenting symptoms in adults and should be treated symptomatically.   2 marks

One in ten infected mothers may have spontaneous miscarriage.   1 mark

Infected foetuses may develop chronic haemolytic anaemia, nonimmune hydrops foetalis, myocarditis, intrauterine foetal death or still birth.   2 marks

IMPORTANT NOTE

Parvovirus B-19 has single stranded DNA and causes 'slapped cheek'/fifth disease (erythema infectiosum) in childhood. It was called fifth disease because it was 5th pink-red rash – following scarlet fever, measles, rubella and roseola – to be described by physicians.

Periods of increased activity are seen during late summer and early spring, every 3 to 4 years in UK.

Transmission is through respiratory secretions, parenteral and vertical routes. Incubation period is 5 to 10 days. Rash occurs between 1 to 5 days after disappearance of viremia and person is noninfective at the time of symptoms.

IgG usually persists for life after acquiring infection and conveys lasting immunity to further infection.

When intrauterine RBC transfusion is performed in the presence of hydrops and anaemia, foetal survival is between 60 to 80 percent. In the absence of any intervention, it is between 15 to 20 percent.

2. A 32-year-old multigravida woman has had a clot in her leg two years back. She is currently 8 weeks pregnant.

a **What are the risk factors for developing thromboembolism in a pregnant woman?** **(7 marks)**

The risk factors for thromboembolism include pregnancy, high parity and pregnancy related to medical disorders causing increased viscosity of blood. 3 marks

Patient characteristics like obesity, age >35 years, previous h/o VTE, congenital and acquired thrombophilia. 2 marks

Pulmonary thromboembolism is the commonest direct cause of maternal death in UK. 1 mark

Risk is highest in the immediate puerperium, following vaginal delivery. 1 mark

b. **How will this information change your management of the remainder of her pregnancy?** **(13 marks)**

Details of her previous illness, treatment taken and duration of treatment should be enquired. Detailed medical records for the diagnosis should be asked for and the concerned physician should be contacted if possible. The diagnosis of past venous thromboembolism should be assumed if good history of prolonged anticoagulation is available. 1 mark

She has an increased incidence of recurrence in the present pregnancy and the risk is proportional to the reason for previous VTE. 2 marks

She should be offered screening for inherited and acquired thrombophilia if not tested before. Multidisciplinary approach with haematologist should be adopted. 2 marks

If previous VTE was associated with pregnancy, she should be offered antenatal prophylaxis with heparin. The prophylaxis should start as early as possible and continue throughout pregnancy. 1 mark

Low dose aspirin should be added in women with antiphospholipid syndrome. Warfarin should preferably be avoided in the first trimester of pregnancy due to the risk of embryopathy. However, it can be safely used in the second and third trimesters, if so required. Its dosage should be carefully monitored by performing the INR ratio. 1 mark

Immobilisation during pregnancy, labour and the puerperium should be minimised and dehydration should be avoided. She should be encouraged to wear graduated elastic compression stockings (TED) throughout their pregnancy and for 6 to 12 weeks after delivery. 1 mark

At the onset of labour, she should be advised, not to inject any further heparin. If she has accidentally taken heparin within a few hours of delivery, its effect can be reversed by the injection of protamine sulphate. She should be re-assessed by senior anaesthetist, haematologist and obstetrician regarding further dose and timing of heparin.   1 mark

If she has received regional analgesia, LMWH should be withheld until 4 hours after insertion or removal of epidural catheter.   1 mark

Women with previous VTE and no thrombophilia should be offered prophylaxis with low molecular weight heparin (LMWH) for 6 weeks after delivery. In women with identifiable thrombophilia, the duration of postnatal prophylaxis depends on specific thrombophilia and varies from 6 to 12 weeks. In women with high-risk of coagulopathy (APH, PPH, wound haematoma), unfractionated heparin should be used for thromboprophylaxis.   2 marks

Combined oral contraceptives should be avoided. Breastfeeding is safe with LMWH and warfarin.   1 mark

IMPORTANT NOTE

Side effects of heparin include—bleeding from overdose, thrombocytopenia, osteoporosis, alopecia (transient and reversible) hypersensitivity reactions. All are less with LMWH. It does not cross the blood brain barrier and placenta. There is a 2 per cent risk of wound haematoma on heparin.

3. **A 49-year-old woman with heavy periods has an endometrial biopsy as part of investigations. Histopathology shows endometrial hyperplasia.**

   Justify her further investigations and management.

   (20 marks)

The type of hyperplasia must further be ascertained as the malignant potential and treatment is dependent on that.   2 marks

Both exogenous (drugs- tamoxifen) and endogenous (ovarian tumour), sources of estrogens should be excluded on history, examination and ultrasound scan.
                                                                                  2 marks

Simple/cystic hyperplasia has very low malignant potential, hence conservative management is appropriate. Treatment with tranexamic acid and/or mefenemic acid or long-term progesterone should be prescribed for symptom control. If she is inadequately controlled with medical management, hysterectomy is justified.
                                                                                  5marks

Adenomatous/complex hyperplasia has a limited malignant potential. Hysterectomy should be offered as it will identify other endometrial pathology and allow further endometrial sampling. On opting conservative management, six months to yearly follow-up with 3/12 progestogens or Mirena intrauterine device and repeat hysteroscopic-guided endometrial sampling should be offered.
                                                                                  6 marks

Atypical hyperplasia has a very high chance of subsequent development of cancer or coexisting with endometrial cancer. Thus, hysterectomy and bilateral salpingo-oophorectomy should be offered as the treatment of choice.   4 marks

If she has a high BMI, weight loss by appropriate means should be advised to reduce non-ovarian oestrogens.   1 mark

IMPORTANT NOTE

The progress to endometrial cancer is less than one in hundred with cystic hyperplasia, 3 to 4 in a hundred with adenomatous hyperplasia and 22 to 33 in hundred with atypical hyperplasia. In 25 to 50 percent cases, atypical hyperplasia is coexistent with carcinomatous change in the uterus.

4. A couple approaches you for tubal ligation as they have completed their family.

    Outline the briefs of your counselling.   **(20 marks)**

The couple should be put at ease and the reason for their request should be explored. She should not seek sterilisation as a cure for menstrual or sexual dysfunction. Appropriate medical history, any problems with past or current contraception, and their sex life should be discussed. Possibility of desiring more children, breakdown of marriage or situation arising due to death of a child should be gently enquired.   3 marks

They should be informed that the procedure is intended to be permanent with 30 to 80 per cent chances of success of reversal operation, should that be necessary. NHS does not pay for the cost of reversal operations or further fertility procedures like IVF or ICSI.   1 mark

They should be informed about other long-term reversible methods of contraception like LNG-IUS, sub-dermal implants and copper intrauterine contraceptives, along with their advantages, disadvantages and relative failure rates.   3 marks

Both vasectomy and tubal occlusion should be discussed. Tubal occlusion carries a lifetime failure risk of one in 200 while vasectomy carries a lower failure rate in terms of post-procedure pregnancy to one in 2000 and there is less-risk related to the procedure.   2 marks

In case of failure of tubal ligation, the resulting pregnancy may be ectopic and she must seek medical advice if she misses her periods or has abnormal abdominal pain or vaginal bleeding.   2 marks

Information leaflets or other recorded information should be provided which they may be taken away and read before the operation to enable them to make an informed decision. Additional counselling sessions may be arranged for young couples or women with special needs to decrease the incidence of regret later.
                                                                3 marks

If the woman is obese, or has had previous abdominal surgery, she should be informed about the risks of laparoscopy and the chances of requiring laparotomy and if there are problems with laparoscopy. Method of access and tubal occlusion to be used in her case should be explained to her.   2 marks

General anaesthesia is usually required for laparoscopic tubal ligation and is a day case procedure. It is not associated with heavier or abnormal bleeding subsequently but few women may experience abdominal pain and psychosexual morbidity.   2 marks

The surgery is commonly performed in the early follicular period and effective contraception should be prescribed till that time.   2 marks

IMPORTANT NOTE

Oral contraceptives are the commonest type of contraception used in UK followed by condoms. Method failure rates per 100 women years of use for common contraceptives are:

Combined pill, LNG-IUS	–	*0.1*
Copper IUD	–	*0.7*
Tubal sterilisation	–	*0.13*
Vasectomy	–	*0.01*
Male and female condoms	–	*4-8*
Emergency c		

Time allowed: 1.45 hours   *MM: 80*

1. A 37-year-old woman conceives following infertility treatment. A scan at 10 weeks shows quadruplets. **(7, 13 marks)**
   a. What are the issues involved in counselling her for foetal reduction?
   b. Discuss the available options for foetal reduction in this pregnancy.

2. A 22-year-old primigravida with no other complications is found to have haemoglobin of 7.8 g/dl at 28 weeks. **(10, 10 marks)**
   a. What investigations would you advise her and how will you diagnose her condition based on these tests?
   b. How will you treat her?

3. Enumerate the precautions that you will ensure for safe laparoscopic entry into the abdomen. **(20 marks)**

4. A 32-year-old woman was found to have bilateral chocolate cysts on diagnostic laparoscopy. She has been trying to conceive for the past 4 years. Discuss the relevant issues. **(20 marks)**

1. **A 37-year-old woman conceives following infertility treatment. A scan at 10 weeks shows quadruplets.**

a. **What are the issues involved in counselling her for foetal reduction?**
(7 marks)

Careful history including ease of conception, parity, and nature of treatment for infertility should be enquired.   1 mark

Both the partners should preferably be present at the time of counselling.
1 mark

The options include nonintervention, selective termination or termination of pregnancy.   1 mark

Couple's moral and religious stance on the subject should be taken into consideration.   1 mark

Appropriate doses of Anti-D should be administered if Rh-negative.   1 mark

Reduction to a twin pregnancy produces the best chances for the remaining babies. Remainder of pregnancy is managed similar to naturally occurring twins.   1 mark

Couples may experience feeling of guilt and opportunities for continued counselling should be offered.   1 mark

b. **Discuss the available options for foetal reduction in this pregnancy.**
(13 marks)

Non-intervention; Advantage is that it is totally natural.   1 mark

There is a high chance of loss of all foetuses which may be unacceptable to this woman. Possibility of prolonged hospital stay, higher incidence of preterm births and its sequelae like cerebral palsy should be discussed. Huge financial and psychological impact of multiple births on the family unit may be unacceptable. Referral to equipped centre with facilities for neonatal intensive care may be required.   3 marks

Termination of pregnancy may be acceptable in women with secondary infertility, to minimise the impact on the rest of the family.   1 mark

Multifoetal pregnancy reduction (MFPR) may be offered between 8 to 13 weeks.
1 mark

Early multifoetal pregnancy reduction is an outpatient procedure done under ultrasound guidance. An ovum pick-up needle is used to enter the sac and the foetal heart. For a 6 to 7 weeks foetus, the foetal heart may be punctured with the needle and potassium chloride may not be required. For 8 weeks and beyond 0.5 to 1.5 cc of 10 percent potassium chloride solution is injected in the foetal heart. Care is taken not to accidentally puncture the adjacent sac(s).   2 marks

Installation of 0.5-1.5 ml of potassium chloride within foetal thorax by trans abdominal approach is the most favoured option. For late foetal reductions nuchal translucency should be measured in all embryos. Embryos having significant risk of aneuploidies or monoamniotic twins are selected for reduction. In the absence of detectable anomalies, choice is based on ease of approach. Embryos close to cervix are avoided. The technical success rate is close to 100 percent.   3 marks

There is a chance of spontaneous loss of an embryo adding to the risk of losing the remaining embryos. After 13 weeks, the chance of spontaneous loss is small. A small theoretical risk of infectious necrosis and DIC remain. Procedure related pregnancy loss rates vary with number of foetuses reduced and is 5 to 10 percent. There is a higher chance of prematurity and foetal growth restriction as compared to twin conception but the outcome is overall better than quadruplet pregnancy.
2 marks

IMPORTANT NOTE

Mean gestational age to which quadruplets reduced to twin pregnancy may continue is 35 weeks.

Triplet to twins is 36 weeks.

Pentaplet to twin is 34+5.

Hexaplet to twin is 33+6.

MFPR is done in late first trimester and mainly reduces the number of foetuses. Selective termination is termination of a mal/developed foetus after the first trimester.

4. A 22-year-old primigravida with no other complications is found to have haemoglobin of 7.8 g/dl at 28 weeks.

a. What investigations would you advise her and how will you diagnose her condition based on these tests? **(10 marks)**

Ethnicity, family history of anaemia and dietary history along with abnormal bleeding from anybody site should be enquired on history. 1 mark

Full blood count with red cell indices; MCV (mean corpuscular volume), MCH (mean cell haemoglobin) and MCHC (mean cell haemoglobin concentration), peripheral smear, serum B-12 and folate levels, screening tests for sickle cell and thalassemia trait should be performed. 2 marks

Serum iron, total iron binding capacity (TIBC) and TIBC saturation should be ordered. Serum iron <12µmol/l and TIBC saturation of <15 percent indicate iron deficiency. 2 marks

Haemoglobin electrophoresis will rule out sickle cell disease, β-thalassaemia and other haemoglobinopathies. A α and β thalassemia trait and disease may be suspected by finding a low MCV, a low MCH, and a normal MCHC. Diagnosis is confirmed by raised concentrations of HbA_2 and HbF in β thalassemia and by globin chain synthesis studies. Father of the foetus may be offered testing in case of positive result as it may also have implications for all future pregnancies. 2 marks

Bone marrow aspiration will help to detect aplastic anaemia. Folate deficiency causes a macrocytic anaemia with megaloblastic changes in bone marrow. MCV is high and serum and red cell folate are low. 2 marks

If history suggests, urine and stool should be tested for haematuria and occult blood. 1 mark

b. How will you treat her? **(10 marks)**

Dietary improvements should be suggested under supervision of a dietician. Tea, coffee and chocolate may inhibit iron absorption and should be minimised. 2 marks

Oral iron supplementation with 100 mg elemental iron should be started and effect of therapy monitored by reticulocyte count 2 weeks later. Vitamin C supplement (orange juice) may help to increase absorption and utilisation. 2 marks

5 mg/day Folate is appropriate for those with established folate deficiency. 1 mark

Oral and parentral iron is contraindicated in thalassemia. Blood transfusions, splenectomy and iron chelation therapy may be required to decrease iron overload in thalassemia major and resistant cases.   2 marks

If anaemia does not respond to oral iron and folate, intramuscular folate may be given. Parentral iron may be required if there are problems with compliance or absorption. Iron sucrose can be safely combined with erythropoietin injections 4000 units subcutaneously weekly, to expedite the rise in haemoglobin if delivery is imminent. Blood transfusion may be thus be averted prior to delivery.
                                                                         3 marks

IMPORTANT NOTE

Iron deficiency is the commonest cause of anaemia in pregnancy followed by Folate deficiency. Haemolytic anaemia, sickle cell disease, thalassemia and hereditary spherocytosis are other causes for anaemia.

Haemoglobin levels below 10.5 g/dl are considered abnormal in pregnancy.

Serum ferritin provides assessment into iron stores and if it is less than 12 µg/l iron therapy should be started.

The increased demands for iron are met by increased intestinal absorption in pregnancy.

MCV is the first index to become abnormal. Serum iron and TIBC fall in normal pregnancy.

3. Enumerate the precautions that you will ensure for safe laparoscopic entry into the abdomen. (20 marks)

Adequately trained and experienced operator, well-maintained equipment and theatre staff is known to decrease overall complication rates during laparoscopy.

3 marks

Each patient should be analysed to identify her risk of bowel adhesion. Palmer's point on left hypogastrium should be utilised, after excluding splenomegaly to visualize the periumbilical area in women at high-risk for bowel adhesions. 2 marks

Preoperatively the bladder should be emptied and abdomen palpated for surface landmarks and abnormal masses. Position of the umbilicus may be variable and iliac crests should instead be used to mark the level of aortic bifurcation. 2 marks

In lean women, entry in Trendelenburg position should be avoided. The horizontal position for all women is currently recommended. 2 marks

The veress needle should be checked for sharpness, spring action and patency, to allow free flow of gas. 1 mark

The umbilicus should be elevated mechanically during insertion of the veress needle to increase the distance between abdominal wall and great vessels. Further insertion should stop once peritoneal cavity is entered. Do not swing the veress needle under the peritoneum. 3 marks

Tests (saline aspiration, gas flow-pressure readings) to confirm the intraperitoneal position of veress should be performed. 2 marks

For adequate distension of abdominal cavity, CO_2 should be insufflated to 25 mmHg until all trocars are inserted and lowered to 12 to 15 mmHg only after insertion. The primary trocar should be inserted through the base of the umbilicus and a 360° survey should be performed to exclude bowel or vascular trauma. Direct trocar entry should be avoided in women at high risk of adhesions. 3 marks

The inferior and superior epigastric vessels should be identified prior to insertion of secondary trocars in lower abdomen. 2 marks

IMPORTANT NOTE

The incidence of major bowel injury during laparoscopic entry is 1 in 2500 and that of major vascular injury is 1 in 5000.

4. A 32-year-old woman was found to have bilateral chocolate cysts on diagnostic laparoscopy. She has been trying to conceive for the past 4 years. Discuss the relevant issues. **(20 marks)**

Endometriosis may be the cause for her infertility. The choice of treatment depends upon several factors including previous treatment, the nature and severity of symptoms, size of cysts, and grade of endometriosis.   3 marks

She should be asked to prioritise her concerns between pain and infertility and treatment initiated accordingly. If infertility is the prime concern, investigations should be commenced for the same.   2 marks

Tubal patency, sperm count and ovulation need to be checked. She should be advised for smoking cessation, cervical screening if due, rubella status and preconception folic acid supplementation.   3 marks

Non-steroidal anti-inflammatory drugs may help in reducing the pain associated with endometriosis. There is no role for medical therapy with hormonal drugs in the treatment of endometriosis infertility.   2 marks

Laparoscopic ablation of all the disease deposits results in higher pregnancy rates. Laparoscopic drainage of the cysts followed by stripping or fulguration of the cyst lining is the procedure of choice. It conserves enough ovarian tissue even when the cysts are large. Simultaneous ablation of all disease deposits result in higher pregnancy rates. If necessary, the ureters should be catheterised prior to surgery.   3 marks

If extensive bowel or bladder adhesions are encountered, laparotomy may become necessary.   1 mark

The use of GnRh agonists prior to or after surgery needs to be individualised. If the cysts are large and leave no room for safe insertion of the laparoscope, preoperative depot GnRh agonists can be employed for three months to shrink the cysts. Postoperatively one should proceed to ovulation induction in the every next cycle and use of medical therapy is to be discouraged.   3 marks

Need for assisted conception depends on her findings. If required super ovulation with GnRH analogues and IUI offer better prognosis. If she has severe endometriosis, referral to a specialist centre for further treatment should be done. All efforts should be made to put her in touch with support groups.   3 marks

IMPORTANT NOTE

The American Fertility Society's scoring system to classify endometriosis is:

Peritoneum

Endometrial deposits	< 1 cm	1–3 cm	>3 cm
Score	1	2	3
Adhesions	Filmy	Dense with partial obliteration of pouch of douglas	Dense with complete obliteration of pouch
Score	1	2	3

Ovary

Endometrial deposits	< 1 cm	1–3 cm	>3 cm
Right score	2	4	6
Left score	2	4	6
Adhesions	Filmy	Dense with partial enclosure of ovary	Dense with complete enclosure of ovary
Right score	2	4	6
Left score	2	4	6

Tube

Endometriosis	< 1 cm	>1 cm	Tube occluded
Right score	2	4	6
Left score	2	4	6
Adhesions	Filmy	Dense with tube distorted	Dense with tube occluded
Right score	2	4	6
Left score	2	4	6

Stage I–mild 1–5

Stage II–moderate 6–15

Stage III–severe 16–30

Stage IV–extensive 31–54

Time allowed: 1.45 hours   *MM 80*

1. A 19-year-old primigravida wishes to discuss pain relief during labour.
           (12, 8 marks)
   a. What are the options available to her?
   b. She wishes to know more about epidural analgesia. What are the contraindications and side effects?

2. The routine 18 weeks scan in a 33-year-old primigravida has shown the presence of echogenic bowel.   (9, 11 marks)
   a. What are the implications of this finding?
   b. How will this finding alter your subsequent care?

3. A 28-year-old woman seeks frequent medical attention for recurrent urinary infections. She is not pregnant and wishes to know the reason for this problem.   (6, 9, 5 marks)
   a. What history and examination would you elicit?
   b. Enumerate the investigations that may be required by her?
   c. How will you treat her?

4. A mother brings her seven and a half year old daughter to your clinic. She is anxious about the breast development in the child.   (10, 10 marks)
   a. On examination you find presence of pubic hair. How will you investigate her?
   b. How will you manage her?

1. A 19-year-old primigravida wishes to discuss pain relief during labour.

a. What are the options available to her? (12 marks)

Presence of a supporting companion during labour and antenatal preparedness of the mother by breathing exercises and antenatal classes help to decrease fear of labour and may decrease the requirement of analgesia. 1 mark

She should be informed that non-pharmacological methods like hypnosis, acupuncture, transcutaneous electrical nerve stimulation (TENS), and audio analgesia may be used in the motivated subject. It may have uncertain efficacy in unmotivated subjects. 1 mark

Nitrous oxide (Entonox-mixture of 50 percent nitrous oxide and 50 percent oxygen) is very popular, self administered, intermittent inhalation analgesia. She has to inhale from the mask, at the first feel of contraction. Moderate pain relief is established 20 to 30 seconds later. It is not very successful in women having mask phobia and in un-cooperative women. 1 mark

Narcotic analgesics like pethidine are given as intramuscular injections (100–150 mg) at the onset of active labour. It is combined with an anti-emetic to offset the side effect of vomiting. It has moderate efficacy, with onset of relief within 10 to 15 minutes and lasting 3 to 4 hours. Its depressive effect on foetus is greatest 2 to 3 hours after maternal administration and least in less than 1 hour or more than 6 hours. It may lead to reduced variability on CTG. The paediatrician should be informed of its use. The effect may be reversed by naloxone given IM to the foetus immediately after birth. 1 mark

Pentazocine does not affect the foetal heart rate but may cause hallucinations and no pain relief in up to 40 percent women. 1 mark

Patient controlled analgesia involves an infusion of analgesic drug like pethidine or pentazocine administered intravenously. The rate of infusion is controlled by the patient through an infusion pump. 1 mark

Epidural block remains the favoured option as it provides complete pain relief. It is an invasive procedure and requires the presence of skilled personnel. 1 mark

Spinal block employs injection of local anaesthetic into subarachnoid space. It is primarily used for second stage procedures like operative vaginal delivery or removal of retained placenta or CS. 1 mark

Pudendal nerve block is injection of local anaesthetic agents like lignocaine in lateral wall of vagina. Used prior to operative vaginal delivery. 1 mark

Para-cervical nerve block is useful for short-term pain relief during the first stage of labour. Foetal bradycardia and marked vasoconstriction can occur because of inadvertent administration in uterine artery. 1 mark

Local infiltration of perineum by lignocaine is effective in reducing the pain due to episiotomy. 1 mark

Information leaflets and contact addresses of hospital antenatal classes should be provided to her. 1 mark

b. She wishes to know more about epidural analgesia. What are the contraindications and side effects? (8 marks)

It involves injection of anaesthetic drug (0.25% bupivacaine and fentanyl) into extradural space in the midline in lateral or sitting position. 1 mark

Adequate circulatory preloading with Hartmann's solution is given to limit any fall in blood pressure. 1 mark

The catheter is usually sited at the onset of active labour and regular top ups are required every 2 to 3 hours. 1 mark

She will feel the uterine contractions but they are not painful. There is a slight reduction in lower abdominal muscle tone which may decrease maternal expulsive efforts causing a slight prolongation of second stage of labour and increase in operative interference. 1 mark

Absolute contraindications of epidural include—refused maternal permission, sepsis in lumbosacral region, conditions predisposing to coagulopathy (severe pre- eclampsia, placental abruption, prolonged retention of products of conception, and thrombocytopenia), use of anticoagulants (except LMWH), severe maternal hypotension and active substantial haemorrhage. Progressive neurological disease is a relative contraindication. 2 marks

Complications of epidural are: Bloody tap, dural punctures (causing headaches), sympathetic block (causing fall in blood pressure- give 5 mg ephedrine if fall is more than 20 mmHg), total spinal block (causing cardiovascular and respiratory collapse) and partial blocks. Retention of urine post delivery due to delayed return of bladder sensations is common. 2 marks

IMPORTANT NOTE

During the first stage of labour, nerves from T_{10}-L should be blocked and S_2–S_5 during the second stage.

Epidural space is between duramater and bony-vertebral canal bound by ligamentum flavum and posterior ligament of the vertebrae.

2. The routine 18 weeks scan in a 33-year-old primigravida has shown the presence of echogenic bowel.

a. What are the implications of this finding? **(9 marks)**

Foetal bowel is considered hyperechogenic when its echogenicity is grossly similar to or greater than that of surrounding bone (foetal iliac crest) regardless of the shape of the echogenic mass in the same machine settings. 1 mark

Its presence is considered a soft marker for trisomy 21. Soft markers are minor ultrasonographic features which may be present in normal foetuses, but have been found in association with abnormal karyotypes. 2 marks

It can be a physiological variant in 67 percent cases. 2 marks

It may be associated with an increased risk of cystic fibrosis, meconium ileus, cytomegalovirus (CMV) infection, adverse foetal outcome such as intrauterine growth restriction and foetal death. 3 marks

Finding a hyperechogenic bowel on ultrasound may be associated with foetal necrotizing enterocolitis after birth and therefore warrants careful investigations. 1 mark

b. How will it alter your subsequent care? **(11 marks)**

Blood samples from mother and father should be tested for DNA mutation analysis for cystic fibrosis. CMV IgM should be tested in maternal blood. 2 marks

Amniocentesis for foetal karyotyping and detection of aneuploidies should be offered in the presence of other soft markers or suspicious serum screening. 2 marks

In the absence of paternal blood samples, DNA mutation analysis for cystic fibrosis can be done from amniotic fluid. Risks associated with amniocentesis should be explained to the mother. 1 mark

High levels of parental anxiety associated with such findings should be acknowledged and expert counselling arranged for if so desired. 1 mark

Even in the absence of any detectable abnormality, remainder of the pregnancy should be supervised by 3 to 4 weekly scans for early detection of growth restriction. Careful search for other ultrasonographic anomalies should be made and if required, woman may be referred to a centre of expertise for the same. 3 marks

Termination of pregnancy option may be offered if foetus is found to be affected by Down's syndrome or cystic fibrosis.   1 mark

Infant may be subjected to immunoreactive trypsin assay and sweat testing to confirm the absence of cystic fibrosis if no testing has been done in parents.
                                                                         1 mark

IMPORTANT NOTE

D F 508 is the commonest mutation causing cystic fibrosis in UK white population.

Echogenic bowel is easily confused with calcifications associated with foetal infection, bowel obstruction/perforation/meconium peritonitis.

Maternal age more than 35 years is an independent risk factor and karyotyping should be offered to such women with echogenic bowel in the absence of any other abnormality.

3. **A 28-year-old woman seeks frequent medical attention for recurrent urinary infections. She is not pregnant and wishes to know the reason for this problem.**

a. **What history and examination would you elicit?** **(6 marks)**

A detailed history of urinary complaints, frequency and duration of illness, and any precipitating factor like menstruation ors sexual activity should be noted.   1 mark

History of diabetes or SLE in self or family should be enquired. Tuberculosis should be kept in mind if she is of Asian origin or has a history of travelling to these areas.   2 marks

Previous records should be checked to note the abnormality in urinary examination.   1 mark

A general physical examination and abdominal examination to look for anaemia and enlarged lymph nodes should be made. Inspection to rule out vulvo-vaginal candidiasis and inflammation around urethral meatus should be made. A pelvic examination should exclude a pelvic mass, large urinary residue and cystocoele.
                                                                         2 marks

b. **Enumerate the investigations that may be required by her?** **(9 marks)**

A clean catch midstream urinary (MSU) sample should be sent for microscopy and culture. Specific cultures, depending on history may be required for tuberculosis or schistosomiasis.   1 mark

A GTT should be done to look for diabetes.   1 mark

Baseline renal functions should be checked in a long-standing problem and with evidence of upper renal tract involvement.   1 mark

An abdominal ultrasound and TVS should be performed to look for pelvic masses compressing urinary tract (ovarian cysts, big fibroids), bladder and ureteric diverticulae, post void urinary residual volume. Both kidneys and urinary tract should be visualised for pressure effects, hydronephrosis, calculi and bladder diverticuli.   2 marks

An Intravenous urogram may be required to visualise the anatomy in select cases. If no abnormality is detected urodynamics should be offered to allow detection of vesico-uretric reflux, urethral pressure profile and pressure flow studies. 2 marks

Bladder cystoscopy and if required directed biopsy should be undertaken to rule out intravesical pathology like bladder calculi, diverticulae, polyps, trigonitis, interstitial cystitis and/or neoplasms.   2 marks

c. How will you treat her?   **(5 marks)**

Management should be directed towards treatment of underlying pathology.

1 mark

General advice on personal hygiene, regular voiding and adequate fluid intake should be given. Cranberry juice is effective in reducing adhesiveness of bacteria to the urinary tract.   2 marks

Specific antibiotics should be added after culture reports. Urinary culture should be repeated after 2 weeks to check the effectiveness of treatment. If no specific cause is identified, long-term low dose prophylactic antibiotics like norfloxacin, cephalosporin or trimethoprim should be added along with a urinary antiseptic.

2 marks

4. A mother brings her seven and a half year old daughter to your clinic. She is anxious about the breast development in the child.

a. On examination you find presence of pubic hair. How will you investigate her? **(10 marks)**

Take history to note any abnormal signs and family history of precocious puberty.

1mark

Undertake a general physical examination to note height, weight and Tanner stages of development.

1 mark

75 per cent of precocity in girls is idiopathic but life threatening neoplasms of ovary, CNS and adrenal must be ruled out.

1 mark

Serum estradiol, FSH, LH, T_3, T_4, TSH, prolactin, testosterone, DHEAS and HCG should be checked.

4 marks

An X-ray of wrist joint for skeletal maturation should be done. Repeat 6 monthly if required.

1 mark

Abdominal ultrasound and/or CT to evaluate ovarian, uterine or adrenal gland enlargement is important. Brain imaging studies like CT or MRI should be done if indicated.

2 marks

b. How will you manage the child? **(10 marks)**

Extensive counselling should be arranged for the girl and her family as social stigma and decreased height due to premature closure of epiphyseal growth centres are usually the main concerns.

3 marks

Multidisciplinary approach is advisable.

1 mark

Management depends on the cause, and the extent of precocious signs and also if the cause requires surgical removal.

2 marks

Gn-RH agonists can be used to suppress the changes if they are causing psychological embarrassment. Depot monthly injections are used for 3 to 6 months till the median age of puberty. Longer use may predispose to osteoporosis.

3 marks

The drug of choice for McCune –Albright syndrome is testolactone that blocks estrogen production.

1 mark

IMPORTANT NOTE

Secondary sexual characteristics before age eight years or menarche before age nine years constitutes precocious puberty.

Thelarche precedes the onset of adrenarche (development of axillary and pubic hair) and menarche (onset of menstruation) at the time of puberty. The average age of puberty is declining and is specific for native populations.

Precocious puberty should be subdivided into two classifications:

1. ***GnRH dependent:** (True/central/complete).There is premature maturation of hypothalamic-pituitary-ovarian axis, usually due to unknown reasons. This is the most common.*
2. ***GnRH independent:** (incomplete/pseudo/peripheral). This is independent of hypothalamic-pituitary control. The most common reason is an estrogen secreting ovarian tumor, 60 percent are granulosa cell tumors. McCune-Albright syndrome is a rare cause.*

McCune-Albright syndrome is a triad of café-au-lait spots, fibrous dysplasia and cysts of skull and long bones.

1. A 30-year-old parous woman at 28 weeks of pregnancy presents at labour ward with high grade fever and loin pain. Her urine dipstick test for nitrites is positive. **(12, 8 marks)**
   a. What will be your immediate management?
   b. Describe your plan of care for her.

2. A 31-year-old woman attends for ante-partum visit at 26 weeks. An opportunistic cervical smear done during the visit shows severe dyskaryosis. **(20 marks)**
   a. Discuss the management of her abnormal smear and possible implications for pregnancy.

3. A 22-year-old woman presents at your clinic complaining of foul smelling discharge. She had a normal vaginal delivery one week back at your hospital. On examination you found a retained swab in her vagina. She is furious at the development and threatens to sue the hospital. **(11, 9 marks)**
   a. Outline your immediate management.
   b. What are the risk management issues?

4. A 15-year-old sexually active woman comes to you for contraceptive advice. How will you counsel her? **(20 marks)**

1. **A 30-year-old parous woman at 28 weeks of pregnancy presents at labour ward with high grade fever and loin pain. Her urine dipstick test for nitrites is positive.**

a. **What will be your immediate management?** (12 marks)

She should be hospitalized. The most likely diagnosis is pyelonephritis. 1 mark

Ascertain a history of previous such episodes. Women with diabetes and on steroid therapy are more vulnerable to developing pyelonephritis. 1 mark

Monitor her pulse, temperature, blood pressure, intake and urinary output record. Hypotension and tachycardia are ominous signs. 1 mark

Send full blood count, serum urea, creatinine, electrolytes, 24 hours creatinine clearance, and blood cultures. A mid-stream urine sample (MSU) for culture should be sent. 2 marks

May need to arrange ultrasound KUB to exclude hydronephrosis, congenital abnormalities and calculi. 1 mark

Chest X-ray with abdominal shield should be done to exclude pneumonia if there is tachypnoea or chest signs. 1 mark

Commence IV antibiotics without waiting for the culture results. IV amoxi-clav (1g 6 h) or cephalosporin's (cefuroxime-750 mg 8 h) are usually the first choice. In allergic /resistant cases an amino glycoside such as gentamicin may be added. IV antibiotics should be continued till the patient is afebrile for 24 hours. After that oral preparations, it should be continued for at least 2 weeks. 2 marks

Appropriate intravenous fluids to maintain urinary output >30 ml/hour should be given. 1 mark

Antiemetics may be required initially, if vomiting is severe. 1 mark

Acetaminophen should be used to reduce pyrexia. 1 mark

b. **Describe your plan of care for her.** (8 marks)

Renal functions and blood chemistry should be re-assessed after 48 hours and then periodically depending on severity. 1 mark

Multidisciplinary approach with involvement of nephrologists and urologists is required if there is no clinical improvement within 72 hours. One in four women have a transient but significant decline in renal and haematological parameters suggested by thrombocytopenia, anaemia, DIC, haemolysis, perinephric abscess, septicemic shock and ARDS. 2 marks

Risk of preterm delivery and low birth weight babies increase significantly. Antenatal steroids should be added and foetal well-being monitored periodically by NST and ultrasound studies. 2 marks

She can be discharged, if she has been afebrile for 24 to 48 hours. She should be advised to increase her oral intake of clear fluids. 1 mark

Follow-up antenatal visit should be arranged after 3 weeks and repeat urine culture should be taken. 1 mark

Postpartum intravenous urography should be offered to women having history of recurrent UTI in pregnancy. 1 mark

IMPORTANT NOTE

4 to 7 per cent pregnant women have asymptomatic bacteriuria, of whom up to 40 per cent will develop symptomatic urinary tract infection in pregnancy and two per cent develop pyelonephritis.

80 to 90 per cent of bacteriuria is due to E. coli and is related to sexual intercourse related ascending infection from perineum.

Significant bacteriuria occurs with colony counts more than 105 ml of MSU specimen.

Screening and treatment of asymptomatic bacteriuria will prevent 70 per cent of all cases of pyelonephritis.

In pregnancy, renal clearance is increased by 40 percent and GRF by 50 per cent but there is a decreased clearance of theophylline. Serum creatinine and BUN values decrease.

2. **A 31-year-old woman attends for ante-partum visit at 26 weeks. An opportunistic cervical smear done during this visit shows severe dyskaryosis.**

a. **Discuss the management of her abnormal smear and possible implications for pregnancy.** **(20 marks)**

Progressive potential of severe dyskaryosis is 20 per cent at 10 years and 80 to 90 per cent women will have CIN II-III at the time of diagnosis of an abnormal cytological smear. This is the same as in non-pregnant women. **2 marks**

She should be urgently referred for colposcopy and seen within 2 weeks. **1 mark**

HPV testing may be performed and if negative the chances of progression to squamous cell carcinoma are low. **1 mark**

Further management depends on colposcopic and biopsy findings. **1 mark**

A colposcopically directed biopsy is required for histo-pathological confirmation. These biopsies are safe and are 99 per cent accurate in pregnancy. **1 mark**

Associated bleeding due to pregnancy induced hyperaemia can usually be controlled by vaginal packing, silver nitrate or haemostatic sutures. **1 mark**

If biopsy confirms invasion, an MRI should be done to see the extent of lesion, and deliver by caesarean section as soon as possible in order to start definitive treatment by radiotherapy. The foetal outcome may be secondary in the light of invasive carcinoma. **3 marks**

Course of steroids should be administered antenatally before delivery. **1 mark**

Option of Caesarean werthiems hysterectomy can be utilised in a referral centre after adequate counselling. **1 mark**

If biopsy shows a non-invasive lesion (CIN I, II, III), treatment should be deferred till after delivery. She should then be followed up 6 to 12 weeks after delivery for a "See and treat policy". If any suspicious findings are present after colposcopy, a repeat biopsy is taken otherwise, she is kept under follow-up. **3 marks**

If CIN I is identified on this biopsy, simply repeating the cervical smears after 6 months of delivery is adequate. Conservative ablative methods like cryotherapy and cold coagulation or laser vaporisation may be used in such women. **2 marks**

If CIN II or III is identified, woman must be allowed to make an informed decision regarding the mode of treatment. Excisional methods like LLETZ (large loop excision of transformation zone), NETZ (needle diathermy excision) are the mainstay of treatment. Look and treat policy should be adopted 6 to 12 weeks after delivery.   3 marks

IMPORTANT NOTE

All women between the ages of 25 and 49 years should have cervical screening with Pap smear every 3 years, and between 50 and 64 years, every 5 years. The results should normally be made available in writing from the GP within 6 weeks. HPV screening should be performed in women with abnormal smears.

Cancer of the cervix is the second most common cancer worldwide, after cancer breast in women under 35 years.

3. **A 22-year-old woman presents at your clinic complaining of foul smelling discharge. She had a normal vaginal delivery one week back at your hospital. On examination you found a retained swab in her vagina. She is furious at the development and threatens to sue the hospital.**

a. **Outline your immediate management.**   **(11 marks)**

The retained swab should be removed and a high vaginal swab should be taken for culture and sensitivity.   2 marks

Her vital signs such as pulse, blood pressure and temperature should be checked.   1 mark

A complete blood count should be checked to assess her white cell count. There is a possibility of gram-negative and anaerobic septicaemia which can present with low blood pressure, tachycardia with or without high temperature.   2 marks

If symptomatic, other than the offensive odour, she should be covered with appropriate antibiotics for gram-negative and anaerobic organisms like a combination of metronidazole with third generation cephalosporin or quinolones.   2 marks

She should be patiently counselled that her symptoms had resulted from a retained swab. She should be informed that it is a rare occurrence and since it has been removed now it will not lead to any further complications. She should also be explained that to prevent such an occurrence the swabs should be counted by the nurse/midwife prior to and after any surgical procedure. Occasionally, there may be an error in counting which can result in this condition.   4 marks

b. **What are the risk management issues?**   **(9 marks)**

A senior obstetric team member available should preferably counsel this patient.   2 marks

Empathy and apology should be offered on behalf of the hospital.   1 marks

Appropriate incident reporting forms should be filled and all concerned personnel should be informed of the incident.   2 marks

If she still wishes to sue the hospital, she should be supplied with the necessary forms and procedural documents.   2 marks

A follow-up visit should be arranged for checking the HVS result and prescribing appropriate antibiotics and to dispel any further doubts.   2 marks

4. A 15-year-old sexually active woman comes to you for contraceptive advice. How will you counsel her? (20 marks)

Establish a good rapport with her by being gentle, objective and non-judgemental.

1 mark

Identify the reason for this visit, and other sexual and mental health issues involved. Elicit her education status, social and financial support, and previous sexual, menstrual and reproductive history along with alcohol, cigarette and drug abuse. 2 marks

Discuss the emotional and physical implications of sexual activity, including the risks of pregnancy and sexually transmitted infections. 2 marks

Assess her competence to consent to treatment by her ability to understand the information provided, to weigh up the risks and benefits, and to express her own wishes. 2 marks

If she is assessed competent, proper documentation of her being 'Fraser ruling competent' (that she understands the advice, will have or continue to have sex, she has been advised to inform her parents, this is in her best interest) should be made in her case notes. 2 marks

Acknowledge her right to confidentiality from healthcare professionals and provide information leaflets mentioning the risks and benefits of various contraceptive choices, sexual health and other lifestyle issues, and appropriate website addresses. Make her aware of the law in relation sexual activity with a young person and that her consent would be sought if information is to be shared or confidentiality breached. However, consent is not essential if the disclosure is justified. 3 marks

She may use combined oral contraceptives (COC), the progestogen only pill (POP), and the progestogen only implant and injections. All medical contraindications should be ruled out and general advice regarding the risks and benefits of individual methods should be imparted to her. Give her time and support to make an informed choice. The effect of hormonal contraception on Bone mineral density is superseded by the effect of factors including exercise, nutrition, calcium intake, and smoking. 2 marks

Use of condoms and safe sex practices should be promoted at all times for prevention of STIs and HIV. 2 marks

Explore the possibility of exploitation and abuse by enquiring whether the relationship is mutually agreed. Child protection agencies should be contacted if there are suspicious circumstances. 2 marks

Enquire whether she wants you to inform her GP. Encourage discussion with a parent, caretaker or another trusted adult. Respect any refusal.   1 mark

Assess any additional counselling or support needs. Arrange appropriate follow-up after 3 months or whenever they develop any problems with the contraception.
                                                                                            1 mark

IMPORTANT NOTE

The legal age of consent to sexual activity in Scotland, England and Wales is 16 years. Sexual activity under the age of 16 years is an offence even if consensual or both parties are aged less than 16 years. The offence is committed by the person, who has sexual intercourse or other sexual activity with the person less than 16 years – not by the person aged under 16 herself.

The legal guidance issued in 1986 after the Gillick case states that health care professionals are justified in giving confidential contraceptive advice and treatment to under 16s provided that (Gillick's Competence)—
- *She/he understands the advice provided and its implications.*
- *Her/his mental or physical health would otherwise be likely to suffer and so provision of advice or treatment is in their best interest.*
- *When it is believed that there is a risk to the health, safety or welfare of a young person or others which is so serious as to outweigh the young person's right to privacy, they should follow agreed child protection protocols.*

FRASER guidelines issued in 1985 during the Gillick's case hearing are:

- *The young person understands the health professional's advice;*
- *The health professional cannot persuade the young person to inform his/her parent or allow the doctor to inform the parents that he/she is seeking contraceptive advice.*
- *The young person is very likely to begin or continue having intercourse with or without contraceptive treatment.*
- *Unless he or she receives contraceptive advice or treatment, the young person's physical or mental health or both are likely to suffer.*
- *The young person's best interests require the health professional to give contraceptive advice, treatment or both without parental consent.*

SEXUAL offences Act 2003 states that

A person is not guilty of aiding, abetting or counselling a sexual offence against a child where they are acting for the purpose of:
- *Protecting a child from pregnancy or sexually transmitted infection.*
- *Protecting the physical safety of a child.*
- *Promoting a child's emotional well-being by the giving of advice*

Over 25 percent of young people aged under 16 years are sexually active but as a group are least likely to use contraception including condoms. Three out of four parents with a child under 18 years feel that young people should have access to confidential contraceptive advice (BMRB survey, 2004). Provision of such services does not lead to earlier sexual activity.

1. a. Discuss the various tests that can be used to screen for the presence of Down's syndrome in pregnancy. **(10, 10 marks)**
   b. You have been asked to see a 36-year-old woman to tell her about her screen positive status and to inform her about amniocentesis. Give the briefs of your counselling.

2. During a routine antenatal visit, a 26-year-old parous woman reveals that she had developed severe depression after the birth of her last child.

   Outline your approach towards her. **(20 marks)**

3. A 20-year-old woman has been referred to you by the GP. She is anxious on account of the death of her mother due to metastatic ovarian cancer and is worried that she may die of the same. Her elder sister is on treatment with Tamoxifen for breast cancer.
   What are the issues involved? **(20 marks)**

4. A 15-year-old girl comes to your clinic accompanied by her mother and reveals that she has not started to menstruate yet. **(13, 7 marks)**
   a. Outline the briefs of your history and examination.
   b. How will you investigate her?

1. a. Discuss the various tests that can be used to screen for the presence of Down's syndrome in pregnancy. (10 marks)

Integrated test gives the best performance provided good quality nuchal translucency (NT) measurement is available and woman is ready to wait until the 2nd trimester for results. It integrates NT +PAPP-A (pregnancy associated plasma protein A) measured at 10 completed weeks and Quadruple test done at 14 to 20 weeks into a single test result. At 85 per cent detection rate (DR), the FPR is only 1.2 per cent, which makes it cost-effective. 2 marks

Serum integrated test is potentially the best, if NT measurements are not available. It uses only serum markers: PAPP-A at 10 weeks +Quadruple test at 14 to 20 weeks. At 85 per cent, DR it has a False positive rate (FPR) of 2.7 per cent. 1 mark

Combined test is for women who require screening in first trimester and understand the implications of doing so. Combines NT measurement +β hCG + PAPP-A at 10 weeks. At 85 per cent DR, the FPR is 6.1 per cent. 1 mark

Quadruple test is a second trimester test for women who attend late. It measures Alpha-fetoprotein (AFP) + unconjugated estriol+ β-hCG + inhibin-A. At 85 percent DR, it has FPR of 6.2 percent. 1 mark

Triple test is a second trimester test. Measures AFP+μ E_3 + β-hCG at 14 to 20 weeks. At DR of 85 per cent, FPR is 9.3 percent, it is not recommended. 1 mark

Double test is a second trimester test. Measures AFP+ β-hCG. FPR is 13.1 percent and is not recommended. 1 mark

Nuchal translucency measurement is done at 11 to 13 completed weeks and has FPR of 20 per cent if used alone. 1 mark

Before measuring the serum levels of markers, gestational age should be assessed accurately. Most accurate dating is by an early dating scan done between 8 to 12 weeks + 6 days. Screening performance of first trimester and second trimester tests is similar. Screening in individual trimesters is much less effective than integrating serial measurements from both trimesters into a single test. 1mark

Routine anomaly scan at 20 weeks will pick up soft markers of Down's Syndrome like increased nuchal fold thickness, wide inter-orbital distance, absence of nasal bone, echogenic bowel and congenital cardiac defects will also pick up downs babies. However, Amniocentesis is the Gold standard confirmatory test. 1 mark

b. **You have been asked to see a 36-year-old woman to tell her about her screen positive status and to inform her about amniocentesis. Give the briefs of your counselling.** **(10 marks)**

The aim of antenatal screening for Down's syndrome (DS) is to offer women, during pregnancy, a screening test which can identify those women at higher risk of having an affected child. In your situation, this pregnancy may be at a slightly higher chance of having a down syndrome baby. This is what is meant by screen positive. 1 mark

This test in itself does not mean that this baby is decidedly going to be affected by Down syndrome. It just has shown an increased chance of being so and now we need to confirm the status by a diagnostic test like amniocentesis. 1 mark

Amniocentesis is removal of small amount of amniotic fluid from the mother's womb for karyotyping. It is the commonest invasive pre-natal diagnostic procedure performed in UK and has high patient acceptability. 1 mark

It is performed trans abdominally between 15 to 18 weeks under ultrasound guidance. The idea is to prevent the needle from injuring the baby so as to not hurt her. 1 mark

A rapid test result (PCR) would be available within 72 hours for Down's syndrome and a few aneuploidies but a full negative culture report takes 2 to 3 weeks. Fluorescent in situ hybridisation (FISH) will provide rapid testing (within a day) for chromosome 21, 18, 13, X and Y. Moreover, it circumvents the problem of failed cultures. About 0.5 per cent of cultures fail and maternal contamination leads to diagnostic difficulties in < 0.2 percent. 2 marks

Complications of the procedure are foetal loss (0.5-1% risk), preterm labour and delivery, lung hypoplasia, respiratory distress, postural limb deformities, foetal trauma by needle, risk of alloimmunisation in rheuses negative women (15%), and bloody tap (0.5%). 2 marks

Appropriate doses of Anti D would be added if required. 1 mark

Information leaflets should be provided and a follow-up date arranged before she goes home. 1 mark

IMPORTANT NOTE

To ensure uniformity and consistency in reporting, a risk cut-off of 1 in 250 at term has been adopted. All screening tests take maternal age into account.

UK Down's syndrome screening programme has adopted a new benchmark for screening tests, to be achieved by 1st April 2007, i.e. tests should have a detection rate (DR) of at least 75 per cent with a false positive rate (FPR) of <3 per cent. SURUSS provided the required evidence leading to this policy. The earlier performance standard for the tests was DR > 60 per cent with FPR 5 per cent or less to be achieved by April 2005.

*SURUSS: First and second trimester antenatal screening for Down's syndrome; the results of **serum, urine and routine ultrasound screening study**. SURUSS does not support retaining double/triple test/NT measurements on their own as each would lead to many more invasive diagnostic tests without increasing the proportion of DS pregnancies detected.*

In DS pregnancy, μ E_3 and AFP are lower while hCG, PAPP-A and inhibin A are elevated.

95 per cent of non-disjunction trisomy 21 is maternal in origin and the risk increases with increase in maternal age. Likelihood of foetus with DS at 35 years is 1:140, at 40 years 1:45, at 45 years 1:15.

Translocation trisomy (inherited/de novo) is not associated with maternal age.

Cost to UK NHS is estimated to be £ 15,300 per affected pregnancy detected by integrated test, £16,800 by quadruple test, and £ 19,000 by combined test.

2. **During a routine antenatal visit a 26-year-old parous woman reveals that she had developed severe depression after the birth of her last child.**

   Outline your approach towards her. **(20 marks)**

This woman should be considered high risk for developing depression in the postpartum period as a previous episode is an indicator and risk factor for the same. 1 mark

Assess her current status by eliciting detailed past and family psychiatric history, current medications, social and financial support. Her relationship with her parents, partner and other children should be explored. 1 mark

Encourage her to reveal any stressful life events regarding her occupation, finances, loss in the family or friends. Any suicidal thoughts or tendency for self-harm should be enquired directly. 1 mark

Symptoms of depression like increased anxiety, weepiness, insomnia, decreased self-worth and poor self-esteem should be enquired. Antenatal depression increases her chances of having postpartum depression. 1 mark

Thyroid function test should be checked as mild hypothyroidism may be associated with this condition. 1 mark

Explanation and reassurance about her condition should be provided sympathetically. One in ten women experience some form of postnatal depressive illness. 1 mark

DHA (Decosahexaenoic acid) supplementation from the second trimester till lactation may help to reduce depression. 1 mark

Multidisciplinary approach by early referral to psychiatrist and, clinical psychologist for assessment should be adopted. Community based midwife and general practitioner should be involved in her care during the post-natal period. She should be advised to get in touch with the local health visitor and the importance of psychological support should be emphasised to the partner. Cognitive behaviour therapy may be offered. 3 marks

Contact numbers of voluntary support organisations like MAMA (Meet a Mum), and the association for post-natal illness should be provided to her. 1 mark

If symptomatic, consideration should be given to start psychotropic drugs. Lithium is contraindicated in first trimester and cardiac scan should be offered at 22 weeks if she continues to take lithium. Tricyclic antidepressants are safe to use during pregnancy. 2 marks

Vigilance should be maintained to look for any abnormal behaviour, abnormal concerns about baby or self, in the post-natal period. In severe cases, she should be transferred to dedicated mother and baby units along with the infant. Electroconvulsive therapy (ECT) is not contraindicated for severe cases. Care should be taken to ensure baby's safety. 3 marks

Prophylaxis with antidepressants can be considered in the post-natal period but as the peak incidence is around 6 weeks postpartum, long-term community based care should be arranged. 1 mark

Encourage breastfeeding as it enhances woman's self image. If she is on psychotropic medication infant should be watched for signs of toxicity. Continue antidepressants for at least 6 months. Most tricyclics and sertraline are safe during lactation. Individual assessment regarding risk vs. benefit of breastfeeding should be made after discussion with the woman. 2 marks

Risk of recurrence depends on severity of depression and varies from 25 to 50 per cent. 1 mark

IMPORTANT NOTE

Incidence of maternity blues—50 per cent

Incidence of post-natal depression—10 to 15 per cent

Incidence of puerperal psychosis—0.2 per cent

According to DSM -1V criteria (American), postpartum depression is diagnosed when the woman experiences at least 5 of the following symptoms for over 2 weeks;

Depressed mood, anhedonia, significant changes in weight or appetite, insomnia or hypersomnia, psychomotor agitation or retardation, fatigue, inappropriate guilt or feeling of worthlessness, impaired concentration or indecisiveness and recurrent thoughts of death or suicide.

3. **A 20-year-old woman has been referred to you by the GP. She is anxious on account of the death of her mother due to metastatic ovarian cancer and is worried that she may die of the same. Her elder sister is on treatment with Tamoxifen for breast cancer.**

   What are the issues involved? (20 marks)

Women with a first degree relative with breast cancer have a two-fold risk of development of breast cancer compared to the normal population. Two first degree relatives increase this risk to four-fold due to genetic inheritance. 3 marks

An abnormality in the BRCA-1 gene increases susceptibility to both breast and ovarian cancer. This gene is localised to the long arm of chromosome 17 and is transmitted by autosomal dominant inheritance. Over half the women who inherit this gene from either the mother or the father will develop breast cancer by 50 years of age. The lifetime risk of breast cancer in such patients is 80 per cent. 3 marks

The lifetime risk of ovarian cancer in the general population is 1 in 70. If a first degree relative has ovarian cancer, the risk is 5 per cent and if two first degree relatives have it the risk is 7 per cent. The hereditary syndromes described, are a site specific ovarian cancer syndrome and breast ovarian cancer syndrome. 3 marks

A second gene BRCA-2 gene is located on chromosome 13. Its presence confers a high risk for early development of breast cancer but is associated with only a small increase in ovarian cancer. 2 marks

Hence, this woman can be offered screening for both breast and ovarian cancers. Her options are to have breast screening with regular monthly self-breast examination with yearly clinical examinations. Yearly mammography should be started earlier, i.e. from 30 years onwards. 3 marks

Ovarian screening is done by yearly pelvic examination, trans-vaginal ultrasound coupled with colour Doppler and six monthly CA 125 levels from the age of 25 years. 3 marks

She should be counselled that she can undergo screening for mutated BRCA 1 and 2 genes. A negative result will be reassuring. However, if positive, it may warrant prophylactic oophorectomy after she completes her family and even prophylactic mastectomy. The decision to undertake this test must be made by the patient depending on her psychological concern. 3 marks

IMPORTANT NOTE

BRCA 1 increases the lifetime risk of breast cancer by up to 80 per cent and of ovarian cancer by up to 50 per cent.

BRCA2 increases the breast cancer risk by 80 per cent and of ovarian cancer by 15 per cent. It also increases the male breast cancer risk by 5 to 6 per cent.

4. A 15-year-old girl comes to your clinic accompanied by her mother and reveals that she has not started to menstruate yet.

a. Outline the briefs of your history and examination. **(13 marks)**

The commonest cause of primary amenorrhoea is constitutional delay. 1 mark

A history of delayed menarche or polycystic ovarian syndrome (PCOS) in mother or sisters is relevant and may suggest a similar trend in the girl. 1 mark

Past history of any prolonged illness, trauma to skull, radiotherapy, chemotherapy, or medications like steroids or anti-hypertensives that may have interfered with pituitary function, should be enquired. It is important to enquire about features suggestive of intracranial lesions, like headaches, and visual field defects. 2 marks

The order and age of development of breasts, axillary and pubic hair should be enquired to determine her development phase. Excessive sporting activity and recent weight loss may cause hypothalamic amenorrhoea. 2 marks

She should be taken into confidence and enquiry made into any family or school stresses, parental expectations and self image. This is best achieved in the absence of mother in the room. History of substance abuse and drugs should be gently elicited. 2 marks

During her examination, the height, weight and body mass index (BMI) should be calculated. A BMI of more than 18 is usually required for initiation of bleeding.
1 mark

Secondary sexual characteristics should be examined to note her Tanner's staging. Short height, with widely spaced nipples, wide carrying angle and webbed neck may suggest Turner's syndrome. Appropriate height with evidence of obesity, acne and hirsutism suggest PCO. A tall girl with good breast development and scanty pubic hair may indicate androgen insensitivity. 2 marks

Galactorrhoea and thyroid enlargement should be excluded. 1 mark

Inspection of the external genitalia should be performed to exclude an imperforate hymen. A per vaginal examination is not indicated. 1 mark

b. How will you investigate her? **(7 marks)**

Presence or absence of uterus should be confirmed by a pelvic ultrasound scan.
1 mark

If her **secondary sexual characters are present**, and she has a uterus, she should be reassured about constitutional delays and advised to wait for another year.
1 mark

Thyroid stimulating hormone (TSH), serum prolactin, β-hCG and progesterone challenge test should be advised if indicated by history.   1 mark

Absence of uterus in presence of breast development suggests either mullerian agenesis (Mayer-Rokitansky) or the presence of Y chromosome. Thus, testosterone levels and karyotyping should be done. 46XX with testosterone in normal female range suggests mullerian agenesis. 46XY with high testosterone suggests androgen insensitivity. An XO in karyotype suggests Turner's syndrome with likelihood of early ovarian failure.   2 marks

If **secondary sexual characters are absent**, investigations and further management should be guided by her history.

Presence of uterus rules out a Y chromosome. Baseline FSH and LH should be measured. High FSH implies ovarian failure whereas low levels show hypothalamic pituitary failure.   1 mark

Absence of the uterus with absent breast development may indicate gonadal dysgenesis. Gonadal biopsy may be required to diagnose rare enzyme deficiencies.   1 mark

IMPORTANT NOTE

Failure of development of secondary sexual characteristics by age 14 and failure to menstruate by 16 years, in the presence of secondary sexual characters, should be investigated.

Time allowed: 1.45 hours   *MM 80*

1. A 30-year-old primigravida presents at 32 weeks gestation with generalised itching but no skin rash.   (6, 3, 11 marks)
   a. How will you confirm the diagnosis?
   b. What are the risks associated with her condition?
   c. How will you monitor and manage her pregnancy?

2. Mrs Emily, 24/40, is carrying twins and has just had her scan done for foetal biometry. The radiographer seemed concerned as there seems to be significant discrepancy in the growth and estimated weight of the two babies.   (7, 3, 10 marks)
   a. What is the likely diagnosis and how will you confirm it?
   b. What are the management options?
   c. Three days later, a repeat scan shows intrauterine demise of one twin. How will you manage the rest of her pregnancy?

3. A 75-year-old woman has intense itching in her vulva.   (14, 6 marks)
   a. She clinically appears to be suffering from lichen sclerosus. Discuss her management.
   b. Enumerate the complications that may arise out of her condition.

4. A 52-year-old postmenopausal woman complains of hot flushes. She is on treatment with Tamoxifen for breast cancer and wishes to start HRT. How will you counsel her?   (20 marks)

1. **A 30-year-old primigravida presents at 32 weeks gestation with generalised itching but no skin rash.**

a. **How will you confirm the diagnosis?** (6 marks)

The most likely diagnosis is obstetric cholestasis (OC or intrahepatic cholestasis of pregnancy). 1 mark

It is a diagnosis of exclusion. A history of onset of pruritis from second trimester onwards in the absence of rash and altered liver functions is significant. Family history may be found in one-third of the cases. 2 marks

Sleep deprivation, jaundice, (pale stools and dark urine) and steatorrhoea may be associated symptoms. Liver function tests may reveal mild increase in bilirubin, alkaline phosphatase, gamma-glutamyl transpeptidase and total bile acids. There is usually a 2 to 3 fold increase in transaminases (ALT being most sensitive) and up to 100-fold increase in primary bile acids (cholic acid and chenodeoxycholic acid). Pregnancy specific range for transaminases should be taken for reference. In the presence of normal bile salt levels, other hepatic pathology should be looked for. In the presence of persistent pruritis and normal liver function, the tests should be repeated weekly. 2 marks

Liver ultrasound and viral serology (hepatitis A, B, C, EBV, and CMV) should be done to exclude other causes of deranged liver functions and itching. 1 mark

b. **What are the risks associated with her condition?** (3 marks)

Once a diagnosis of OC is made the woman should be counselled concerning the foetal risks like possible preterm delivery, meconium stained liquor, intrapartum foetal distress, intrauterine foetal death and foetal intracranial haemorrhages. 2 marks

Mother is more prone to get vitamin K mal/absorption. Risk of PPH increases at the time of delivery. 1 mark

c. **How will you monitor and manage her pregnancy?** (11 marks)

Foetal well-being should be monitored closely by serial ultrasound scans to check foetal growth, liquor volume, and Doppler umbilical artery blood flow studies. 1 mark

Liver function tests and prothrombin time should be checked weekly. 1 mark

Frequency of antenatal visits should be determined by the severity of condition. 1 mark

Cool baths, bicarbonate washes and topical emollients are helpful in mild cases. Chlorpheniramine at bed time may help to relieve pruritis. Ursodeoxycholic acid to decrease the total bile acid levels is not licensed for use in pregnancy.   1 mark

Cholestiramine may be effective in some women. S-adenosylmethionine (SAM), guar gum, and activated charcoal have no role.   1 mark

Tab vitamin K 10 g oral every day should be commenced after 36 weeks and continued till delivery.   1 mark

Offer to deliver her at 38 weeks as risk of foetal death may increase after 36 weeks. If condition aggravates, antenatal steroids should be given before 34 weeks. Risk of induction and possible caesarean section should be explained to the mother.   2 marks

Labour should be closely monitored by electronic foetal monitoring and precautions taken to prevent PPH. Neonate should receive injection vitamin K at birth. After delivery, pruritis may take 1 to 2 weeks for resolution.   1 mark

Repeat LFT's after 10 to 14 days to check resolution. If required biliary tract ultrasound for gallstones should be performed.   1 mark

Risk of recurrence in subsequent pregnancies is high 50 to 60 percent. Standard oestrogen containing oral contraceptives should be avoided but low dose preparations may be advised under supervision.   1 mark

IMPORTANT NOTE

Incidence of OC is higher in women of Asian origin especially Indian and Pakistani women. In pregnancy upper limit of bilirubin and gamma- glutamyl transferase is 15 to 20 percent lower.

2. **Mrs. Emily, 24/40, is carrying twins and has just had her scan done for foetal biometry. The radiographer seemed concerned as there seems to be significant discrepancy in the growth and estimated weight of the two babies.**

a. **What is the likely diagnosis and how will you confirm it?** **(7 marks)**

Twin-to-twin discordance with transfusion (TTTS) is the most likely diagnosis.

1 mark

History and examination of the mother may be consistent with excessive growth of the uterine fundus suggesting polyhydramnios. 1 mark

An obstetric ultrasound is the most important diagnostic tool. It may confirm monochorionicity (single placental mass and concordant foetal sex) and show evidence of discordant foetal biometry (difference of more than 15 per cent in estimated weights), and/or structural malformations. 2 mark

There would be near anhydramnios in the sac of the growth deficient twin with a small urinary bladder. 1 mark

The recipient twin may have evidence of hydrops, ascitis, ventricular hypertrophy or congestive cardiac failure along with a full urinary bladder indicating severe TTTS. There may be polyhydramnios in the amniotic sac. 1 mark

Umbilical artery Doppler may show a difference of more than 0.4 in the umbilical artery systolic/diastolic ratios and presence of a vascular anastomosis between the co-twins. 1 mark

b. **What are the management options?** **(3 marks)**

Refer to a tertiary care, foetal diagnosis and treatment unit. 1 mark

Amnioreduction and laser membrane septostomy may result in prolongation of pregnancy. 1 mark

Ultrasound guided umbilical cord occlusion using bipolar diathermy may be used to selectively coagulate the offending vessel in order to allow at least one twin to survive. 1 mark

c. **Three days later, a repeat scan shows intrauterine demise of one twin. How will you manage the rest of her pregnancy?** **(10 marks)**

In monochorionic pregnancies, the mortality and morbidity of surviving twin is greatly increased. One in four foetuses will have neurological damage, including cerebral palsy, porencephaly, hydrocephalus and cerebral infarction. Renal cortical necrosis may occur. 1 mark

Offer bereavement counselling to the mother and family.   1 mark

DIC (disseminated intravascular coagulation) in the mother can be a complication *in utero* demise and immediate and weekly coagulation studies should be carried out.   1 mark

Investigations to check uteroplacental insufficiency and hostile uterine environment should be carried out as they could be a threat to the surviving twin as well.   1 mark

The surviving twin should be serially assessed by using cardiotocography and ultrasound (biophysical profile, biometry).   1 mark

Antenatal corticosteroids should be given to mother to prevent neonatal respiratory distress in surviving twin in case of premature delivery.   1 mark

The psychological status of woman and her preferences should be taken into account before deciding about the time of delivery. Risks of prematurity versus the risk of *in utero* damage must be balanced. Expectant management may be adopted especially when >24 hours have elapsed since the event.   1 mark

Caesarean section is generally the preferred route if preterm delivery is indicated. Delivery may be delayed up to 37 weeks in dichorionic pregnancy in the absence of any maternal or foetal compromise.   1 mark

After delivery the newborn should be assessed by cranial ultrasound and MRI in case of any abnormality. Baby may require prolonged neurodevelop/mental follow-up by pediatricians.   1 mark

GP and social worker should be informed at the time of discharge to offer extended support and counselling to the couple.   1 mark

IMPORTANT NOTE

Another name of TTTS is Feto- foetal transfusion syndrome (FFTS) or twin oligohydramnios- polyhydramnios sequence (TOPS).

It affects 10 to 15 per cent of all monochorionic pregnancies with a higher incidence in monochorionic-diamniotic twins rather than monochorionic- monoamniotic pregnancies. The placentas mostly have a unidirectional artery to vein anastomoses.

The mortality rate is very high i.e. 60 to 100 per cent for the twins. Mortality with TTTS increases with earlier diagnosis. Survival rates are higher if there is higher number of artery- artery anastomoses between the co-twins

3. A 75-year-old woman has intense itching in her vulva.

a. She clinically appears to be suffering from lichen sclerosus. Discuss her management.   **(14 marks)**

Lichen sclerosus can cause intense pruritis vulvae. It typically causes white "cigarette paper plaque- like" lesions.   1 mark

A biopsy of the lesion is warranted especially if there is a doubt over the diagnosis, or to rule out squamous carcinoma.   1 mark

Since the oetiology is thought to be autoimmune, allergy or genetic predisposition, treatment is with topical steroid cream application and emollients. Milder steroid creams like 1% hydrocortisone may not provide relief of symptoms. Use stronger steroid creams like clobetasol (0.05%), betamethasone or fluocinalone. These can be applied every night during an acute episode and then two to three times a week during remission.   3 marks

During periods of remission weaker steroid creams like hydrocortisone may also be used daily. Some patients may be controlled on emollients alone during remission.   2 marks

Use of oestrogen creams is of no value as there are no oestrogen receptors on the vulval skin.   1 mark

Testosterone creams have been used with good relief of symptoms. However, the testosterone gets absorbed and may cause hirsutism.   1 mark

Local destructive procedures like cryo-cautery or CO_2 laser have no role as they only remove the epidermis and do not treat the underlying changes within the dermis. Healing may be prolonged and may produce more discomfort and distortion.   2 marks

Simple vulvectomy cannot be justified in lichen sclerosus as it often recurs in the excision margins. However, it is justified if hyperkeratotic patches appear or there is a suspicion of malignancy.   2 marks

Patient should be followed up every six monthly to rule out development of vulval cancer.   1 mark

b. Enumerate the complications that may arise out of her condition.
                                                    (6 marks)

It may cause cosmetic concerns, especially if it spreads in extra genital areas also.
                                                    1 mark

Dyspareunia, urinary obstruction, and secondary infection from chronic skin micro ulcerations may happen.   2 marks

Chronic steroid use may cause skin atrophy and secondary infections.   1 mark

Vulval carcinoma can occur in 3 to 5 per cent patients of lichen sclerosus. Squamous hyperplasia or vulval intra-epithelial neoplasia (VIN) have been seen in biopsy specimens adjacent to lichen sclerosus in half the patients. Older age, concomitant infection with Chlamydia, longer duration of lichen sclerosus and evidence of squamous hypertrophy are associated with higher risk of development of VIN.

2 marks

4. A 52-year-old postmenopausal woman complains of hot flushes. She is on treatment with Tamoxifen for breast cancer and wishes to start HRT.

How will you counsel her? **(20 marks)**

HRT is effective for symptomatic relief of menopausal symptoms and its use is justified if symptoms are adversely affecting her quality of life. However, she should be made aware of the risks and allowed to make an informed choice. 2 marks

Details of her complaint, its effect on her quality of life, time since menopause (prophylactic oophorectomy?), expectations from treatment along with family,medical and treatment history should be enquired for a need and risk analysis. 2 marks

Recent bone densitometry, baseline LFT, RFT, TSH may be useful. If her BP is elevated and hot flushes are the quite troublesome, consider ruling out pheochromocytoma. 2 marks

For mildly symptomatic women, lifestyle changes (limit smoking, alcohol, and caffeine intake, and start moderate weight bearing exercises) combined with non-prescription medications includes dietary isoflavones, mineral and calcium supplements and vitamin E may be prescribed. 2 marks

She should avoid black cohosh and soy products. Known triggers for vasomotor symptoms like hot and spicy foods or drinks, hot environment and stress should be avoided. Weight gain should be kept under check. 2 marks

HRT with only estrogens is effective and may even decrease her risk of breast cancer. Therapy should be initiated only after discussions with her oncologist and the type of cancer. Therapy with combined estrogens and progestogens is contraindicated in women with breast cancer. 3 marks

Tibolone is effective in the treatment of hot flushes and may increase the risk of breast cancer but lesser than the risk by combined hormonal preparations.
1 mark

Progestogens such as norethisterone 5 mg/day or megestrol acetate 40 mg/day are effective in the control of hot flushes but may flare progesterone receptor positive breast cancer. 1 mark

Selective serotonin reuptake inhibitors (SSRIs) may be helpful in treating hot flushes and are not contraindicated in breast cancer. Their use may be associated with temporary decrease in libido. 1 mark

Multidisciplinary counselling should be encouraged. Prior to commencement of treatment she should discuss its effect on her condition with her oncologist. Contact numbers of local support groups of menopausal women should be provided.   2 marks

Information leaflets documenting risks and benefits of individual HRT preparations should be provided and follow-up appointment in the menopausal clinic arranged.
                                                                2 marks

Time allowed: 1.45 hours   *MM 80*

1. A 32-year-old woman has been referred to you by the GP with a random blood sugar of 8.3 mmol/l. She is currently 26 weeks pregnant and has no history of diabetes mellitus before.   (15, 5 marks)
   a. Discuss your plan of management in this pregnancy.
   b. How will you supervise and manage her labour?

2. A 20-year-old has tested positive for HIV during her booking investigations.   (10, 10 marks)
   a. How would you proceed further in the next 4 weeks?
   b. She has decided to continue with her pregnancy. Discuss your plan of management.

3. A 32-year-old woman complains of urinary frequency and pain in her lower abdomen while passing urine. The pain is so severe that it leaves her incapacitated for 5 to 10 min. This is third episode in this year and her MSU has always been normal.   (12, 8 marks)
   a. What relevant history, examination and investigations would you like to conduct in order to reach a diagnosis?
   b. Cystoscopy has confirmed interstitial cystitis. How will you treat her?

4. A 28-year-old woman complains of persistent vaginal discharge despite various medications prescribed by her GP.   (4, 11, 5 marks)
   a. What may be the cause of her symptoms?
   b. What will you look for during the initial assessment?
   c. What advice will you give regarding her condition?

1. A 32-year-old woman has been referred to you by the GP with a random blood sugar of 8.3 mmol/l. She is currently 26 weeks pregnant and has no history of diabetes mellitus before.

a. Discuss your plan of management in this pregnancy. **(15 marks)**

One random sample on its own is suggestive but not sufficient for diagnosis of diabetes and formal 2 hours oral GTT should be done after 8 hours of fasting followed by 75 gm glucose load. Further management depends on the result of O-GTT and she should be classified as normal, impaired GTT or gestational diabetes mellitus (GDM). 2 marks

If normal, pregnancy should proceed as per protocol and GTT should be repeated at 28 to 30 weeks of gestation and the situation reviewed. 1 mark

Note BP and body mass index at every visit. Check glycosylated haemoglobin (HbA1c), routine pregnancy investigations and urinalysis. Gestational age should be accurately calculated from first trimester scan. 2 marks

If she has mild degrees of impaired glucose tolerance, she should be reassured as the perinatal outcome is similar to that in healthy population. A timed random glucose sample and urine for glycosuria should be checked at each antenatal visit. 1 mark

Life style and dietary modifications are important. Diet with reduced fat, increased fiber and regulated carbohydrate intake of low glycemic index should be stressed under supervision of a dietician. 35 Kcal/kg+300 Kcal with a diet composition of 40to 50 per cent carbohydrates, 12 to 20 per cent protiens and 30-35 per cent fats is advisable. Total intake should be spread between 3 main meals and 3 snacks. 2 marks

If she is classified as GDM, a multidisciplinary team should be involved in her care. Serial scans may be required to assess foetal growth and liquor volume. Repeat HbA1$_c$ every 6 weeks. Weekly NST should be done from 38 weeks if she is controlled on diet alone and from 32 to 35 weeks if insulin is required. May need more frequent monitoring after 37 weeks. 2 marks

A baseline 24 hours blood sugar profile should be done and repeated serially depending on the severity. Persistent postprandial hyperglycemia (> 7.5-8 mmol/l) or fasting hyperglycemia (> 5.5 mmol/l) despite compliance with diet for a week is an indication for introduction of insulin therapy. Dietary modifications should continue till term in addition to insulin. 1 mark

She should be encouraged to monitor her own blood sugar at home (HBGM) with glucometers, the frequency of monitoring being proportional to derangement in blood sugar. Human actrapid insulin should be preferred with its dose and frequency adjusted by postprandial values. 1 mark

Elective caesarean section may be considered in the presence of mal-presentations, an estimated foetal weight in excess of 4.5 kg, or a history of previous caesarean section. Continue pregnancy till term if good control of diabetes is achieved. Each case should be assessed individually regarding time of induction, if required. Routine inductions at 38 weeks and waiting till 41 weeks have similar CS and shoulder dystocia rates. Encourage breastfeeding after delivery. Ask her to keep a light snack handy while breastfeeding.   2 marks

Progesterone only pills, barriers and low-dose estrogen pills can be prescribed for contraception. Offer her GTT with 75 gm glucose within 6 weeks to 3 months of delivery to assess her status. She should be made aware of the long-term risk of developing NIDDM associated with GDM. Recurrence rate in next pregnancy can be minimized by achieving ideal BMI prior to conception.   1 mark

b. How will you supervise and manage her labour?   **(5 marks)**

Adequate labour analgesia (epidural) should be considered to avoid catecholamine associated hyperglycemia.   1 mark

Labour should be carefully supervised with partograms, CTG and experienced midwifery staff.   1 mark

Women with impaired GTT either do not require insulin during labour or small doses are given using a sliding scale. Those on larger doses of insulin should be managed by insulin infusions as per the labour ward protocol.   1 mark

For frank diabetics and those requiring high doses of insulin in antenatal period infusions of human actrapid insulin 10 units in 100 ml of normal saline should be started at 10 ml/hr using a micro-drip set. Blood sugar should be checked every hour in the other arm. If blood sugar is between 4 to 6 mmol/l, continue the same dose of insulin. If <4 mmol, halve the rate of infusion and if >6 mmol then double the rate of insulin infusion till optimum sugar levels are achieved. Halve the rate of insulin infusion after delivery. In the other arm she should constantly receive 100 ml/hr of 10 per cent dextrose.   2 marks

IMPORTANT NOTE

Women with GDM have 50 per cent risk of developing NIDDM within 10-15 years.

Insulin and glucagons do not cross placenta. There is no increase in brain size in macrosomic fetuses.

AFP, E_3, and HCG values are all lower in diabetics.

GDM is diagnosed if:

1. *After 50 gm glucose load orally, blood sugar level after 1 hour is > 7.8 mmol/l.*
2. *Fasting blood glucose level is > 6.0 mmol/l and 2 hours postprandial value is >9.0 mmol/l (adopted by UK Task force on diabetes) but local guidelines should be followed for treatment purposes.*
3. *The WHO proposes the following criteria after 75 g oral GTT.*

	Normal	Impaired	Frank diabetes
Fasting	< 6 mmol/l	6–7.9 mmol/l	≥ 8 mmol/l and/or
2 hours PP	<9 mmol/l	9–10.9 mmol/l	≥ 11.1 mmol/l

Target plasma glucose levels in pregnancy are:

Before breakfast	*69–90 mg/dl or 4–5 mmol/l*
Before lunch, dinner	*60–105 mg/dl or 4–6 mmol/l*
After meals	*= 120 mg/dl or less than 6.8 mmol/l*
2 AM to 6 AM	*> 60 mg/dl or more than 4 mmol/l*

18 mg = 1mmol of glucose.

2. **A 20-year-old has tested positive for HIV during her booking investigations.**

a. **How would you proceed further in the next 4 weeks?** **(10 marks)**

She should be informed of her HIV result in person, by an appropriately trained health professional. Information leaflets and all information about her subsequent care should be imparted in a non-judgemental manner. 1 mark

Reassure her repeatedly that her confidentiality will be respected. However, all health professionals involved in her care should be aware of her diagnosis. She should be encouraged to inform her seropositive status to her partner but no information should be revealed to people (relatives) who are not at risk of acquiring infection. 2 marks

Contact tracing through an STD clinic should be initiated to identify and treat the index case, and curb further spread. 1 mark

Baseline investigations like complete blood counts including CD4-T lymphocyte count, maternal plasma viral load, serum urea, electrolytes, liver enzymes, blood glucose and lactates should be done and repeated monthly. She should be screened for inflammatory genital infections (*Chlamydia, gonorrhea*, bacterial vaginosis) as soon as possible in pregnancy and at 28 weeks. 1 mark

Screening for syphilis, hepatitis B, and HCV should be offered. 1 mark

Routine pregnancy investigations, detailed ultrasound for foetal anomalies and Down's syndrome screening should be offered. 1 mark

Termination of pregnancy is an option if the women so desires. 1 mark

She should be managed by a multidisciplinary team including an HIV physician, an obstetrician, midwife, pediatrician, psychiatric team and support groups. The case should be reported to National study of HIV in pregnancy and childhood at RCOG. 2 marks

b. **She has decided to continue with her pregnancy. Discuss your plan of management during antenatal period.** **(10 marks)**

She should be informed that interventions such as antiretroviral therapy, elective caesarean section and avoidance of breastfeeding can reduce the incidence of vertical transmission from 25 to 30 per cent to less than 2 per cent. 1 mark

She is likely to be asymptomatic (since she was picked up on screening) with low plasma viral load and CD4 −T lymphocyte count $> 350 \times 10^6/l$. She will require antiretroviral therapy to decrease risk of vertical transmission. 2 marks

Short term antiretroviral therapy (START) from 28 to 32 weeks (oral Ziduvudine 100 mg 5 times a day) should be started and continued intrapartum. If she is at high-risk for preterm delivery (uterine over distension, previous history) therapy should be commenced earlier to achieve undetectable plasma viral load by delivery. 2 marks

Prophylactic steroids to enhance lung maturity should be given if required. 1 mark

Women having symptomatic HIV infection, or low CD4 counts should be advised to commence highly active retroviral therapy (HAART) from 14 to 34 weeks and continued till after delivery. Optimal drug and dose regimen, decision to start, modify or stop retroviral therapy should be determined by an HIV physician in close liaison with the obstetrician and paediatrician. 2 marks

Drug toxicities include cholestasis, GI upsets, fatigue, fever, hepatotoxicity, rashes, glucose intolerance, diabetes, lactic acidosis and mild anaemia. If CD4 counts are $<200\times10^6$/l prophylaxis against *Pneumocystis carinii* pneumonia infection should be given by administering cotrimoxazole and folic acid. 1 mark

Choice of mode of delivery depends on viral load at term. If there is no detectable viral load she can take a trial of labour, otherwise she should be offered elective caesarean section at 39 weeks. 1 mark

IMPORTANT NOTE

HIV is a human retrovirus with double-stranded DNA. Zidovudine; the commonest medicine in use inhibits chain elongation of viral DNA by selectively inhibiting RNA dependent DNA polymerase (viral reverse transcriptase).

Over 80 per cent of mother to child (vertical) transmission occurs late in the 3rd trimester, during labour and at delivery with less than 2 per cent transmission during 1st and 2nd trimesters. Low antenatal CD4-T lymphocyte counts (< 350 × 10^6/l), high maternal plasma viral loads (>20,000 copies/ml), vaginal delivery, duration of membrane rupture >4 hours, chorioamnionitis and preterm labour are associated with increased risk of transmission.

***Intrapartum management** includes Ziduvudine infusion should be started 4 hours prior to skin incision and continued till umbilical cord is clamped. Prophylactic antibiotics should be given to decrease infective morbidity.*

Women who prefer to avoid caesarean section should have their membranes left intact for as long as possible. Foetal scalp electrodes and scalp sampling should be avoided. Ziduvudine infusion (or HAART) should be commenced at onset of

labour and continued till cord is clamped. HIV infection per se is not an indication for electronic foetal monitoring.

Maternal serum samples should be taken for viral loads at delivery. Cord should be clamped as soon as possible and baby should be given bath immediately after birth.

Postpartum management: *She should be advised not to breastfeed the baby as it increases perinatal transmission. Infant should be treated with antiretroviral drugs for 4 to 6 weeks. Polymerase chain reaction (PCR) should be done at birth, 3 weeks, 6 weeks and 6 months to detect infant viral infection.*

Appropriate contraception and use of barriers should be promoted at all times.

Breastfeeding doubles the risk of vertical transmission from 14 to 28 per cent.

3. **A 32-year-old woman complains of urinary frequency and pain in her lower abdomen on passing urine. The pain is so severe that it leaves her incapacitated for 5 to 10 min. This is third episode in this year and her MSU has always been normal.**

a. **What relevant history, examination and investigations would you like to conduct in order to reach a diagnosis?** **(12 marks)**

Elicit a history of flares that correlate with specific events in her life; particularly sexual intercourse. These may be more frequent in the week before her period, intake of foods high in potassium and during the times of stress. 2 marks

Fill in the PUF (pelvic pain/urgency/frequency) questionnaire. A high score is suspicious of interstitial cystitis. 1 mark

Exclude other causes of pelvic pain, dysmenorrhea, dyspareunia and cyclicity. 1 mark

Repeat an MSU to exclude a concurrent urinary infections and vaginitis. Send urinary cultures through a catheter sample. Treat if positive. 3 marks

Intravesical potassium sensitivity test is performed if cultures are negative. Offer diagnostic cystoscopy for positive sensitivity challenge. Presence of classic Hunner's ulcer and/or diffuse glomerulations signify interstitial cystitis. 3 marks

If the potassium sensitivity is negative, consider other etiologies including endometriosis, adhesions, or vulval problems. Diagnostic laparoscopy may be required to see and treat other pelvic pathologies. 2 marks

b. **Cystoscopy has confirmed interstitial cystitis. How will you treat her?** **(8 marks)**

Lifestyle and dietary modifications are an important part of the treatment. She should avoid any known triggers as well as avoid carbonated drinks, alcoholic beverages, and tea, coffee and cranberry juice. 2 marks

Fava beans, onions, tomatoes, tofu, sour cream, yoghurt, chocolate, processed meats, mayonnaise, spicy foods, etc. should likewise be consumed with caution. 1 mark

A multidisciplinary approach involving the urologists is recommended. 2 marks

Pentosan polysulfate is the first line treatment if she is not pregnant. Symptomatic relief may take up to 4 to 6 months. If she does not respond or is pregnant, intravesical heparin may need to be considered. 3 marks

IMPORTANT NOTE

If PUF score is more than 10 to 12, there is an 80 per cent chance that potassium sensitivity test will be positive.

PUF Questionnaire
Pelvic pain and urgency/frequency
Patient Symptom Scale

Please circle the answer that best describes how you feel for each question

	0	1	2	3	4	Symptom score	Bother score
1. How many times do you go to the bathroom during the day?	3–6	7–10	11–14	15–19	20+		
2. a. How many times do you go to the bathroom at night?	0	1	2	3	4+		
b. If you get up at night to go to the bathroom, does it bother you?	Never	Occasionally	Usually	Always			
3. Are you currently sexually active?	YES____ NO____						
4. a. If you are sexually active, do you now or have you ever had pain or symptoms during or after sexual intercourse?	Never	Occasionally	Usually	Always			
b. If you have pain, does it make you avoid sexual intercourse?	Never	Occasionally	Usually	Always			
5. Do you have pain associated with your bladder or in your pelvis (vagina, labia, lower abdomen, urethra, perineum)?	Never	Occasionally	Usually	Always			
6. Do you still have urgency after you go to the bathroom?	Never	Occasionally	Usually	Always			
7. a. If you have pain, is It usually		Mild	Moderate	Severe			
b. Does your pain bother you?	Never	Occasionally	Usually	Always			
8. a. If you have urgency, is it usually		Mild	Moderate	Severe			
b. Does your urgency bother you?	Never	Occasionally	Usually	Always			
Symptom score (1, 2a, 4a, 5, 6, 7a, 8a)							
Bother score (2b, 4b, 7b, 8b)							
Total score (symptom score + bother score) =							

*Total score range is from 1 to 35. A total score of 10–14 = 75 per cent likelihood of positive PST; 15–19 = 79 per cent; 20+ = 94 per cent

4. **A 28-year-old woman complains of persistent vaginal discharge despite various medications given to her by the GP.**

a. **What may be the cause of her symptoms?** **(4 marks)**

A physiological discharge is common during reproductive years. 1 mark

Infections (bacterial vaginosis, candidiasis, trichomoniasis, *Chlamydia trachomatis* and *Neisseria gonorrhoeae*), foreign bodies (forgotten tampons, condoms), cervical polyp and Ectropion, allergy and vary rarely genital tract malignancy would be included in the differential diagnosis. 3 marks

b. **What will you look for during the initial assessment?** **(11 marks)**

Enquire about the colour, amount, duration, consistency, associated smell or itch and the relation of discharge to menstrual cycle. Any recent change in the nature of discharge or sexual partner should be noted. A history of dysuria, dyspareunia, abdominal pain, fever, and abnormal bleeding pattern should be sought. 3 marks

Enquire about her sexual and contraceptive history, menstrual history (pregnancy, post abortion or postpartum), any associated medical conditions (diabetes) and medications (antibiotics, corticosteroids) along with previous treatment history. Compliance with previous medications and side effects like vomiting should be checked. 3 marks

Her risk for sexually transmitted infections (STI) should be assessed. Even in the absence of other factors, recurrent infection refractory to treatment requires laboratory investigations. 1 mark

Palpate abdomen for any pain, inspect vulva for any obvious discharge and vulvitis. 1 mark

A careful speculum examination should be undertaken. Inspect vaginal walls, cervix, foreign bodies and the nature of discharge. High vaginal and endocervical swabs should be taken at this time. Test vaginal pH from lateral vaginal walls using narrow range pH paper. 2 marks

A bimanual pelvic examination should be done to exclude cervical motion tenderness, uterine and adnexal tenderness. 1 mark

c. **What advice will you give regarding her condition?** **(5 marks)**

Provide appropriate treatment with locally available protocols. Vaginal Metronidazole, clindamycin and clotrimazole are usually the first line treatment. For recurrent infection, a weekly dose can be continued for 6 months. 2 marks

She should avoid douching, local irritants, perfumed products, tight fitting synthetic clothing. Alcohol intake with oral metronidazole should be avoided.

1 mark

If diagnosis is an STI, then partner notification and treatment, referral to GUM clinic and specialist advice should be sought. Routine screening and treatment of male partners is not required.

1 mark

Barrier contraceptives may get damaged with vaginal preparations containing clotrimazole. Abstinence or double protection should be advised.

1 mark

IMPORTANT NOTE

Commonest cause of vaginal discharge in young women is physiological.

Commonest infective cause is bacterial vaginosis (not considered a sexually transmitted disease but is associated with early sexual activity and higher number of sexual partners), followed by candidiasis. Commonest bacterial STI is C. trachomatis.

Risk factors to be sought for STI are: age ≤ 25 years, change in sexual partner in the last year; more than one sexual partner in the last year.

High vaginal swab should be sent for:
- *Microscopy and Gram-stain for diagnosis of BV (Amsel's criteria) and Candida spores.*
- *Saline wet microscopy for diagnosis of Trichomonas vaginalis (direct visualization).*
- *Culture in chocolate agar for diagnosis of Neisseria gonorrhoeae (Sabouraud's medium for Candida if microscopy is inconclusive).*
- *Sensitivities: to various locally available treatment regimens.*

Endocervical swab should be sent for culture, ELISA, and NAAT for N. gonorrhoeae and C. trachomatis.

If high vaginal swab cannot be transported immediately to the laboratory, it should be stored at 4° C for less than 48 hours.

ELISA—Enzyme-linked immunosorbent assay.

NAAT—Nucleic acid amplification tests.

BV—Bacterial vaginosis.

Incubation period (in days) of various STIs are:

Neisseria gonorrhoeae	*2–7*
Herpes simplex virus	*2–12*
Trichomonas vaginalis	*4–20*
Chlamydia trachomatis	*7–14*
Treponema pallidium	*14–84*
Human immunodeficiency virus	*30–90*
Human papilloma virus (HPV)	*30–140*
Hepatitis B virus	*45–180*

Time allowed: 1.45 hours   *MM 80*

1. A 30-year-old woman has just had an unexplained stillbirth at term. You are the SpR on duty and have to take consent for post-mortem of the baby. (14, 6 marks)
   a. What are the issues involved?
   b. She is uncomfortable with the idea of having a long cut on her dead baby's body. She wishes to know if anything else can be done.

2. Mrs. Cathie, 35/40, presents at the labour ward with sudden onset of leg oedema and shortness of breath even on lying down. This is her first pregnancy and her pre-natal period has been uneventful so far, except for complains of fatigue during the last visit. (9, 6, 5 marks)
   a. What will be your immediate management?
   b. Her echocardiographic findings suggest cardiomyopathy. What investigations will you order and what trend are they likely to show?
   c. What precautions would you undertake while delivering her?

3. A young woman presents at the accident and emergency complaining of severe abdominal pain and bloating. She has been on injection Menogon for the treatment of infertility. Her last period was 20 days back. (5, 15 marks)
   a. What investigations relevant to her condition will you order?
   b. How will you manage her condition?

4. A 52-year-old caucasian post-menopausal woman has been having backache for the last one month. She is concerned about osteoporosis as her mother had a history of osteoporotic fractures. (7, 13 marks)
   a. What features in her history would put her at a higher risk for osteoporosis?
   b. Her T-score on a DEXA scan is −2.5. How will you manage her?

1. **A 30-year-old woman has just had an unexplained stillbirth at term. You are the SpR on duty and have to take consent for post-mortem of the baby.**

a. **What are the issues involved?** (14 marks)

The women should be handled sympathetically and discussions should preferably take place with both the partners together. 1 mark

A written informed consent from the mother is required for the procedure. Standard perinatal autopsy request and report forms should be filled. 1 mark

Acknowledge that discussions about autopsy are acutely distressing following bereavement and refusal for the same is her right in case of personal or religious objections. 1 mark

She should be informed that autopsy may help to confirm clinical diagnosis, reveal the cause of death, reveal structural anomalies of relevance to the risk of recurrence, provide an estimate to the time of death, identify chronic intrauterine disease (infection, brain damage, etc.) and give information on the complications of treatment. It may be difficult, if not impossible, to advise on the risk of recurrence in a future pregnancy in the absence of autopsy. Even a negative or normal autopsy report is of significance and in some cases no abnormality may be revealed. Sometimes despite tests it is not possible to know the exact cause of death. 3 marks

Consent is required for: 3 marks
1. Post-mortem examination and tissue retention of small samples for histopathological diagnosis. To investigate the molecular basis of unexplained death, foetal DNA should be stored to detect later, the disorders which may later be shown to have genetic basis. DNA extraction requires considerable workload and storage of small amount of foetal tissue is more practical.
2. Use of material (histopathological slides) for teaching, research and possible tissue retention for treatment of others.
3. Organ retention; especially brain and heart for diagnosis of congenital disorders. Whenever possible organs should be reunited with body prior to burial or cremation. When it is not possible, parents can choose either to make their own arrangements or leave it to the hospital to dispose of the organs after investigations have been completed.

Every hospital should have written guidelines for external and radiological examination and for maternal and neonatal investigations in case of perinatal death. Use of foetal tissues and organs can only be carried out if the hospital conforms to Polkinghorne guidelines. 2 marks

Bodies need to be transported from place of delivery/death to a regional centre for specialist autopsy by a perinatal pathologist. Consent should be taken for this transfer. She should be informed about means of transport and when the body will be returned. Written procedures for handling, receipt and return of bodies should exist. Inform the mother that the case will be taken up for discussion at perinatal mortality meeting.   2 marks

Information leaflet should be provided to the parents explaining the purpose of an autopsy, benefits of tissue and organ retention and rights of parents to grant or withhold their agreement. CESDI document "Guide to the post-mortem examination: Brief notes for parents and families who have lost a baby in pregnancy and infancy" should be recommended.   1 mark

b. She is uncomfortable with the idea of having a long cut on her dead baby's body. She wishes to know if anything else can be done.
(6 marks)

Parents who decline perinatal autopsy should be offered limited autopsy.   1 mark

This includes external examination, tissue needle biopsy, body cavity aspiration, imaging (X-ray, ultrasound, MRI), targeted open tissue biopsy and placental biopsy.
2 marks

Post stillbirth karyotyping has a high failure rate. Multiple samples should be collected usually from placenta and full thickness skin biopsies.   2 marks

Specific consent for each component should be taken. It must be stressed that these techniques remain inferior alternatives to full post-mortem with histopathology.   1 mark

2. Mrs. Cathie, 35/40, presents at the labour ward with sudden onset of leg oedema and shortness of breath even on lying down. This is her first pregnancy and her pre-natal period has been uneventful so far, except for complains of fatigue during the last visit.

a. What will be your immediate management? **(9 marks)**

Peripartum cardiomyopathy or pulmonary thromboembolism are the likely diagnosis. (oedema, orthopnoea, fatigue, no previous cardiac history).   1 mark

Admit Mrs. Cathie to HDU. Start pulse oxymetry and oxygen by mask.   1 mark

Get good IV access and withdraw sample for investigations. Put her on fluid restricted, low sodium diet and in propped up position.   1 mark

Obtain obstetric ultrasound and NST.   1 mark

Initiate multidisciplinary management by involving physician and cardiologist.
   1 mark

Reduce after load by reducing the systolic BP to less than 110 mmHg. Calcium channel blockers like amlodepin or nitro-glycerine or hydralazine can be started.
   1 mark

Diuretics should be used with caution as they will reduce the uteroplacental circulation. Digoxin or dobutamine may be required to improve cardiac contractility.   1mark

Anticoagulation prophylaxis with unfractionated heparin should be started.
   1 mark

If she develops pulmonary oedema- positive pressure airway breathing or intubation may be required.   1 mark

b. Her echocardiography suggests changes similar to cardiomyopathy. What investigations will you order and what trend are they likely to show? (6 marks)

FBC- normal, liver function tests-may be elevated if right heart failure involved.
   1 mark

B-type natriuretic peptide, serum creatinine-elevated, Troponin, creatine kinase- normal unless ischaemia.   1 mark

EKG – may reveal atrial fibrillation.   1 mark

Chest X-ray – Cardiomegaly, pulmonary oedema or pleural effusion   1 mark

Echocardiogram- Ejection fraction less than 45 percent, shortening fraction less than 30 percent, dilated left ventricle.   1 mark

c. What precautions would you undertake while delivering her? (5 marks)

Vaginal delivery is preferred and CS is reserved for usual indications.   1 mark

Minimise cardiac work during labour and delivery. Instrumental delivery may be required.   1 mark

Use regional anaesthesia to reduce preload and after load. Start prophylactic antibiotics.   1 mark

If she gets breathless, add low dose beta blockers to her existing medication.
                1 mark

After delivery add diuretics to reduce cardiac work and switch to ACE inhibitors. Switch to low molecular weight heparins followed by warfarin.   1 mark

IMPORTANT NOTE

The diagnostic criteria for peri-partum cardiomyopathy are:
1. *Development of cardiac failure during the last trimester or within 5 months post-partum.*
2. *Absence of identifiable cause for cardiac failure.*
3. *Absence of recognisable heart disease in the past.*
4. *Demonstration of left ventricular systolic dysfunction by echocardiography showing an ejection fraction < 45 percent, shortening fraction<30 percent, left ventricular end- diastolic dimension>2.7cm/m².*

3. A young woman presents at the accident and emergency complaining of severe abdominal pain and bloating. She has been on injection Menogon for the treatment of infertility. Her last period was 20 days back.

a. What investigations relevant to her condition will you order? (5 marks)

The most likely diagnosis is Ovarian Hyperstimulation syndrome.   1 mark

Investigations should include FBC, haematocrit, urea and electrolytes, creatinine, liver function test especially albumin levels, coagulation profile, ultrasound scanning, and chest X-ray.   3 marks

Serum beta HCG to confirm pregnancy.   1 mark

b. How will you manage her condition? (15 marks)

She should be admitted in the hospital and investigated to establish the severity of her condition, preferably under the supervision of a specialist in reproductive medicine.   2 marks

A multidisciplinary approach may be required for her care.   1 mark

Hypovolaemia should be corrected by infusion of Hartmann's solution or normal saline, with added potassium if required. Increasing the oncotic pressure with the use of Human albumin solution is controversial. The use of plasma expanders like hydroxyethyl starch is better than haemaccel which gives a temporary relief.   2 marks

Recent evidence suggests that daily administration of bromocriptine 2.5 mg orally/ per rectally will reduce the levels of vascular endothelial growth factor (VEGF) and reduce third space loss.   1 mark

Thromboprophylaxis with heparin is necessary. Mannitol or dopamine may be required in oliguric patients. Pneumatic compression stockings should be used if patient is confined to bed.   1 mark

Prostaglandin synthetase inhibitors should be avoided for analgesia as they may decrease the renal blood flow.   1 mark

Close monitoring of pulse, respiratory rate, blood pressure, temperature, fluid balance and urinary output should be maintained. Haematological parameters and abdominal girth measurements should be repeated every day initially. An in-dwelling catheter may be required, if the output is low/ difficult to measure or in the presence of voiding difficulties. Additional monitoring with pulse oximetry or admission to intensive care unit will depend on the severity of the condition.   4 marks

Drainage of third space accumulations may be necessary to improve distress and urinary output. Abdominal or pleural paracentesis should be done under ultrasound guidance.   2 marks

Surgical intervention should preferably be avoided but may be required in cases of ovarian torsion or significant intra peritoneal bleeding.   1 mark

IMPORTANT NOTE

A haematocrit greater than 0.48 or sodium level less than 135meq/l, serum potassium more than 5.0mEq/L and creatinine levels more than 1.2mg/dl indicate a need for hospitalisation.

4. **A 52-year-old caucasian postmenopausal woman has been having backache for the last one month. She is concerned about osteoporosis as her mother had a history of osteoporotic fractures.**

a. **What features in her history would put her at a higher risk for osteoporosis?** (7 marks)

Her post-menopausal status, being a caucasian woman and positive family history definitely increase her risk of osteoporosis. 1 mark

Cigarette smoking or excessive use of alcohol may decrease her bone mass. 1 mark

A History of long term medications like corticosteroids, anti-convulsants, heparin, thyroxine or hormones like tamoxifen, depo-progesterone and GnRh analogues may also be relevant. 2 marks

A medical history of disorders like Cushing's, hyperthyroidism, anorexia and eating disorders, thalassemia, premature ovarian failure etc will increase her risk. 2 marks

A diet deficient in vitamin-D and calcium or a history of gastrectomy will also decrease her bone density. 1 marks

b. **Her T-score on a DEXA scan is –2.5. How will you manage her?** (13 marks)

Explain to her that a T- score of –2.5 means that her bone density is 20 to 25 percent lower as compared to a normal person of her age and she is already in the osteoporotic range. At these values, her risk of hip and spinal fracture is 8 to 10 times increased. 2 marks

Lifestyle related risk factors including smoking, alcohol and exercise should be discussed. 2 marks

Advise her to get an X-ray of lumbosacral spine as her backache may be due to compression fractures. Nasal calcitonin is effective to reduce pain associated with such fractures. 2 marks

A multidisciplinary approach with involvement of orthopaedicians/ physiotherapists should be encouraged. 1 mark

Alendronate 70 mg per week or raloxifene 60 mg daily should be added to prevent further bone loss. 1 mark

Consider HRT or ERT (oestrogen replacement therapy). 1 mark

Add calcium 1200 to 1500 mg/day as calcium citrate and vitamin D 400 to 800 mg daily. If she is on ERT, her calcium requirements are less, i.e.1000 to 1200 mg/day.   2 marks

She should be encouraged to start weight bearing exercises and repeat her DEXA scan after 6 to 12 months.   2 marks

IMPORTANT NOTES

Peak bone mass is normally achieved by 30 years and after that there is a loss of 0.4 percent every year. After menopause the loss is accelerated to 2 percent of cortical bone and 5 percent of trabecular bone.

A healthy bone comprises of 75 percent of cortical (outer shell) and 25 percent of trabecular (spongy/inner) bone.

ERT reduces lifetime fracture risk by half and the greatest benefit of HRT is obtained, if started shortly after menopause.

If T-score is between 0.0 and – 0.9, then bone mass is normal.

T-score between –1.0 and –1.4, bone mass is 10 to 15 percent below normal and fracture risk is 2 to 2.5 times.

T-score between –1.5 and –1.9, bone mass is 15 to 20 percent below normal and fracture risk is 3 to 4 times higher.

T-score between –2.0 and –2.4, bone mass is 20 to 25 percent lower and fracture risk is 5 to 7 times greater.

T-score of –2.5 and lower, then bone mass is more than 25 percent lower and fracture risk is 8 to 10 times higher.